To Hayat Barron
with many thanks
and appreciation for
the new energy you
bring to our Children's
Taskforce

5/18/05

What the Professionals are Saying

"An excellent book, both in conception and execution...I've reviewed it as publication nears, and vouch for its accuracy and sensible approach. It's a fine book, far more digestible and useful than The Physicians Desk Reference, or any recent texts on psychopharmacology or psychiatry."

> **—Jonathan O. Cole, M.D.**
> Professor of Psychiatry, Harvard Medical School, Boston
> Senior Consultant McLean Hospital, Belmont

"You don't need to have an MD, or PhD, to understand this book. It is family friendly, practical, and informative. I would strongly recommend this book as an essential reference for all who are caring for a child or adolescent who has been diagnosed with a serious emotional disorder or a mental illness."

> **—Kathleen Considine, M.S.W., L.S.W**
> Affiliate/IFSS Liaison, NAMI New Jersey

"The straight forward discussion 'Should my child be on medication?' speaks clearly and directly to our parents. These issues addressed in Dr. Perrin's book benefit not only the children, but the whole behavioral health care system as well."

> **—Barbara Chayt**
> Special Needs Administrator, Juvenile Justice Commission

Psychiatric
Medications
for Children

A handbook for parents and other professionals who work with children and need to know their medications and understand their parents' perspective. This group includes teachers, guidance counselors, psychologists, as well as other mental health, child welfare, and juvenile justice personnel.

Psychiatric Medications *for* Children

Medication and Treatment for
Children and Youth with Emotional
and Behavioral Challenges

MARK PERRIN, M.D.

The Stillwater Press, Inc.
Stillwater, New Jersey

Psychiatric Medications for Children

Medication and Treatment for Children and Youth with Emotional and Behavioral Challenges

Mark Perrin, M.D.

The Stillwater Press, Inc.
P.O. Box 265, Stillwater, New Jersey 07875-0265

Cover and Book design: Peri Poloni, Knockout Design, www.knockoutbooks.com

Printed by: Book-mart Press, Inc., 2001 Forty Second Street, North Bergen, N.J. 07047

Publisher's Cataloging-in-Publication
(Provided by Quality Books, Inc.)

Perrin, Mark, 1934-
     Psychiatric medications for children : medication and treatment for children and youth with emotional and behavioral challenges / Mark Perrin.
     p. cm.
     Includes bibliographical references and index.
     "A handbook for parents and other professionals who work with children and need to know their medications and understand their parent's perspective. This group includes teachers, guidance counselors, psychologists, as well as other mental health, child welfare, and juvenile justice personnel."
     LCCN 2005901002
     ISBN 0-9716977-1-X

     1. Pediatric psychopharmacology — Popular works. 2. Behavior disorders in children — Chemotherapy — Popular works. I. Title.
     RJ504.7.P47 2005   618.92'8918
               QBI05-200033

This book is dedicated to my family.

*Ursula, my wife, who has selflessly supported me
in all my endeavors and who has enhanced
the clarity of each page.*

*Thomas, Christopher and Nicholas, my sons,
who have taught me much and
inspire me to learn more.*

With love and gratitude.

Acknowledgements

I want to acknowledge and thank those who read the manuscript and provided constructive criticisms and creative contributions:

Jonathan O. Cole, M.D
> Professor of Psychiatry Harvard Medical School, Boston
> Senior Consultant, McLean Hospital, Belmont

Kathleen Considine, M.S.W., L.S.W.
> Affiliate/IFSS Liaison, and Walk Coordinator, NAMI
> New Jersey

Nancy T. Block, M.D., F.A.P.A.
> Past President New Jersey Psychiatric Association

Shannon Brennan
> Mental Health Administrator, Warren County, New Jersey

Catherine Brewster
> CART Coordinator, Warren County, New Jersey

Mary Thiele
> Services Specialist, Division of Youth and Family Services
> Warren and Sussex Counties, New Jersey

For generous assistance in producing the manuscript, and for remarkable patience during its revisions, special thanks are given to:

Carol Deresz
> Administrative Secretary, Department of Human Services,
> Warren County, New Jersey

With Special Recognition of

Sylvia Axelrod

Executive Director of NAMI NEW JERSEY
for her unswerving dedication to persons affected by mental
illness and establishing the NAMI NJ Task Force for Children and
Adolescents in order to better address their needs.

Karen Kubert

Director Department of Human Services, Warren County,
NJ who has been a life-long advocate for children with serious
emotional disorders and has provided them,
and their families, support and assistance.

About the Author

A fter Princeton, Mark Perrin received his M.D. degree from New York University College of Medicine. In his postgraduate residency programs, he chose to focus on the specialties of internal medicine and neurology. As a practicing internist with The Summit (New Jersey) Medical Group, Dr. Perrin developed a particular interest in the biological connections between physical and emotional states. His continuing inter-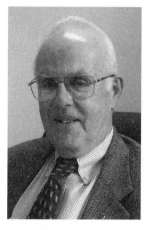est in neurology has led to an active membership in the American Neuropsychiatric Association.

Currently, Dr. Perrin serves as the president of the New Jersey State affiliate of a worldwide organization, The National Alliance for the Mentally Ill (NAMI). He is president of the New Jersey Parents' Caucus and has served on Governor Codey's Mental Health Taskforce Children's Committee. For several years, he chaired the State Mental Health Advisory Board and is currently the chairman of the Warren County Mental Health Board. In his work on the County Case Assessment Resource Team, he oversees children whose emotional and behavioral problems put them at risk of being removed from their homes. Watching these parents struggle to get appropriate mental health services for their children has, he believes, kindled his strong spirit of advocacy.

About New Jersey
Parents' Caucus

The New Jersey Parents' Caucus is an independent not-for-profit organization whose mission is to insure that every family which has children with special emotional and behavioral needs is given an opportunity to play a strong and active role in the development and delivery of appropriate, effective and timely services for all children.

In 1990 a small group of concerned parents formed the New Jersey Parents' Caucus to radically reform the State system delivering services to New Jersey families and children with severe emotional and behavioral needs. The NJPC spearheaded a coalition to change existing policy and to advocate for appropriate services.

This group formulated the "principles of care" which became the foundation upon which a new comprehensive system for children's mental health services was built. This system, now known as the "New Jersey Division of Child Behavioral Health Services" was revolutionary in that the needs of children drive the system and the system partners with parents at all levels from local to State, and at all phases of activity including planning, oversight, and quality assurance.

Principles of Care

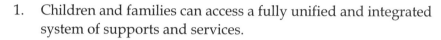

1. Children and families can access a fully unified and integrated system of supports and services.

2. Children and family services are planned and implemented with agency collaboration, coordination, and leadership at all levels (state, county, local).

3. Parents/family members are full partners in all aspects of the process.

4. Children and families receive services from service providers and other professionals who are fully prepared to work as partners with families.

5. Children and families can access "family friendly", culturally compatible services.

6. Children and families can access a full continuum of prevention services, and models that promote healthy development and self sufficiency.

7. Children and families can access a full continuum of intervention services as early as needed, in the least restrictive, most natural environments.

8. The needs of children and families are addressed by systems that engage in ongoing assessments of individual needs as well as overall needs of children and families throughout the state.

9. Children and families can readily access information regarding their own services, as well as the overall performance of system and services.

10. Children and families receive efficient, sufficient, effective and fully funded services.

About NAMI New Jersey

NAMI New Jersey is a statewide organization dedicated to improving the lives of individuals and families who are affected by mental illness.

Affiliate self-help and grassroots advocacy groups are located in every county to offer emotional support, information, advice about treatment, and community resources.

NAMI New Jersey provides:

Education: On a local, state, and national level, NAMI provides education and confronts discrimination through awareness campaigns.

Support: In local self-help groups, caring family members offer emotional support, information, and advice.

Advocacy: On a state and local level NAMI NJ promotes and supports Legislative issues that benefit families and persons affected by serious mental Illness, monitors governmental agencies responsible for the provision of Services and promotes research into the causes and treatment of mental illness.

NAMI New Jersey is the state affiliate of the now worldwide organization founded in 1979 as the National Alliance for the Mentally Ill which works to enhance services and treatment for the more than 15 million Americans living with severe mental illness and their families.

Nationally 225,000 members, more than 1000 local affiliates, and 50 state organizations all work to provide support, education, and to advocate for funding of research, and all the supports necessary to achieve wellness and well-being.

How to Use This Book
"As Easy as One, Two, Three"

⸺⁀

1. First and Foremost — THE MEDICATIONS
Chapter 10   pp 34-99

This book is a ready resource for important information about psychotropic medications, useful to all individuals involved with children and youths who have emotional and behavioral disorders. The basic information about each medication is succinctly organized under section headings: **description, mechanism of action, indications and uses, side effects, monitoring, warnings, what else you need to know.**

2. Second and Still Foremost — PARENTS' CONCERNS
Chapters 1 – 6   pp 4-19

Additional relevant information is presented in the form of general discussions that address the most important concerns of parents and caregivers.

3. Third — INTRODUCTION TO NEUROSCIENCE
Chapters 7 – 9   pp 20-33

Basic science about neurons and the organization of neurons within the brain are included for those who want to know more about how and where medications work. This material is not needed to access the important information about medications. Rather these sections provide context and supplementary material to enhance understanding and interest. Those who grasp the basic principles presented will enter the promising and rapidly expanding world of neuropsychiatry.

Table of Contents

General Purpose

The purpose of this book is to educate and thus empower parents and caregivers. It is very important that parents have access to information about medications in order to understand what they do and why they have been prescribed. Increasing knowledge about psychotropic medications will help in talking with the doctor and developing mutual understanding and cooperation. A parent-professional partnership is most important to ensure that the child receives optimal benefit from treatment.

Chapter 1

About Children's Mental Health Services

The recent Surgeon General's Report* tells us:

One of every 5 children has a diagnosable mental illness.

One in every 10 children has a mental illness severe enough to cause disability, interfere with normal development and requires urgent treatment.

Only one in five children who requires treatment ever receives it.

Of this small fraction of children receiving treatment it remains unknown how many are receiving treatment that is appropriate, effective, and of sufficient duration to be a proven benefit.

The problem of obtaining mental health services for children is compounded by a shortage of child psychiatrists. Furthermore, only a minority of primary care physicians are adequately trained to diagnose children's mental illness. Finally a managed care system that pressures primary care physicians to decrease appointment time, that often disallows visits to specialists, erects multiple barriers in this process of accessing mental health care.

In these difficult times in which the availability and quality of children's mental health care can be unpredictable, parents must be alert and, where necessary, become advocates for their children so that those with emotional and behavioral problems receive the help that they need.

* See appendix P. 101, 102 for Visions and Goals

Chapter 2

General Advice About Treatment

M edication should never be thought of as a magic bullet that will cure the problem. Medication can be a valuable part of, but should never be a substitute for, a thoughtful, holistic treatment plan. A plan needs to identify and appropriately utilize the resources of the individual, family, professionals, and community. Unremitting efforts on the part of all the participants to carry out a well conceived and coordinated plan is necessary for the "recovery" of the child and the well-being of the family.

"Recovery" is not used in the sense that the illness is no longer present, but rather refers to the process of successfully managing the symptoms and behaviors caused by the illness.

A child cannot be blamed for having a biologic disease of the brain, but must learn to accept age appropriate responsibility that this is his/her own problem. Strategies must be developed to manage the disruptive symptoms and prevent them from controlling his/her life. Being in "recovery" is taking personal responsibility, learning how to manage symptoms to create a state of "wellness" with a satisfying and rewarding life.

Through the centuries hundreds of treatments have been created to treat emotional and behavioral disturbances. But those treatments which have been proven to be effective all share four basic components.

- Interpersonal connectivity, attunement, contingent

communication, empathetic listening, really being there with full awareness and open mind free of distractions.

- Connecting right brain emotion to left brain reason and allowing emotional matters to be thought about, evaluated, and thus become more "manageable".

- Providing both support and challenge

- Joint narrative, creating jointly an autobiography of who the child is, what the world is like, and how life can be lived.

1.) **Really Being There**

Therapy takes place within a relationship. The therapist needs to come to where the child is emotionally and mentally to feel what the child is experiencing. Other feelings from the therapist's own personal past are pushed aside so as to be solely attuned to the child. The child gains a needed sense of self by simultaneously feeling his emotion and seeing it in the face and body of the therapist. Thus emotions come to be identified by the child and are accepted as part of him/herself. The opportunity to express emotion without devastating consequences also helps the child to understand that emotions are normal. Such experiences help develop the skills of emotional regulation and self- soothing.

2.) Emotional experiences are centered in the right side of the brain while speech and intellectual reasoning are primarily left brain functions. To achieve emotional regulation these two systems need to be connected. Integration of these functions allows for the greatest flexibility in emotional responses to various situations. Therapists need to facilitate interweaving these functions. Teaching children to recognize emotions, and to develop a vocabulary to describe, think, and talk about emotional responses, is a needed part of education.

3.) Having support and a secure home base give a child the reassurance needed to explore, to meet new challenges, to develop a sense of self-confidence and self-competence. For progressive development, skills achieved are valued and supported, but are combined with encouragement to try a new challenge just beyond the present capability.

4.) All individuals need to create a concept of who they are, where they have come from and where they are going. This narrative is important to the developmental process. Joint story telling with a therapist or parent helps create a self-image and reduces self-doubt. If the child has assimilated misconceptions and has a distorted inaccurate sense of self, the misconceptions need to be therapeutically revisited and reframed in the proper perspective. With the helpful input of new information and new insights, the story of self is then jointly rewritten. Culture, community, and family play an important role in creating a child's sense of self.

In truth, good therapy is much like good parenting. While therapists are trained, most parents do a commendable job with only instinct and learned family traditions. But the parents of children with emotional and behavioral challenges need to learn how they can be the most helpful. Parents need to be open, to try to achieve empathetic understanding. This is critical to confirming the reality of the child's experience and helping him/her to develop knowledge of self. Often however, the pace of modern life and multiple responsibilities makes this impractical on a daily basis. But at important times of emotional crisis, children need their parents to be attuned in order to validate, to be empathetic in order to sooth, and to tolerate in order to contain the crisis. By validating, soothing, and containing, the parent demonstrates to the child the defusing and regulation of emotion. Teaching by example helps the child develop the skills needed for controlling his/her own emotions.

When parents feel pressure, feel they are over-reacting to a situation, or are on the verge of "losing it", they too ought to call "time out". An attempt to connect to the child, and to what is going on, should not be made until control is regained. If a parent is never able to actively listen but rather is overcome by emotions related to their own past experience then help should be sought.

It is important to remember that children learn intuitively from what parents are feeling, thinking and doing. They are far too perceptive to believe what is being said when their parents' behavior and actions are conveying a different message. An effective parent is consistent in what is being felt, said and done. This is hard to accomplish but should always be kept in mind as a goal to strive for.

Chapter 3

Important Questions
For Parents

"Should my child be on medication?" is a difficult question
with which parents often must wrestle. The doctor is able to provide information along with professional judgment, but the ultimate
decision and final responsibility rests with parents.

The decision is made more difficult because in most instances
there is insufficient research about the effects of medications in children. Pharmaceutical corporations are reluctant to assume the high
costs of research and the increased legal liability for the more limited market that children and youth present. Consequently, many
medications do not have the clinical studies required by the Food
and Drug Administration for approved use in children. Lack of
such approval does not mean the medications are without benefit
or are dangerous, but rather that clinical studies for children have
not been done.

Children are not small adults and drug effects cannot be assumed
to be the same as in adults. Biological differences between children and
adults, include differences in body composition of water and fat, rate
of absorption, rate of excretion, and rate of deactivation by the liver.
Side effects of drugs can vary at different ages or between sexes.

What, if any, are the effects of medication on the development of a child's brain? What are the possible long term consequences? These questions remain essentially unanswered. Other questions are only partially answered and can give rise to differing opinions among the experts. More research is needed to answer these very important questions universally raised by parents.

Incomplete knowledge of medication effects engenders caution in their use. However, we also do know that troublesome, sometimes disabling, symptoms or problems left untreated or under treated may later cause more serious and severe consequences as the child develops. Sometimes medication treatment for a disturbing symptom or disruptive behavior can stabilize a child. After stabilization other non-medication treatments may become more effective and permit drugs to be discontinued. Of course in some instances, greater benefit is achieved by continuing the medication. Each child and every situation is unique.

What is being treated? It is important to distinguish **symptoms** from **disorders.** Symptoms are the problematic feelings, ways of functioning, or behavior that are caused by an underlying brain disorder. Parents may bring their children to the doctor because of troublesome symptoms. The doctor takes a history, identifies the symptoms and attempts to diagnose the underlying disorder responsible. Diagnosis is difficult but very important. A correct diagnosis provides an understanding of what to expect over a period of time, what other symptoms could develop, and most importantly indicates which treatments are most likely to be helpful. The younger the child the more difficult it is for the doctor to be certain of the underlying condition. Observation of behavior and symptoms over a significant period of time may be needed before a diagnosis can be made with "certainty". If the diagnosis is tentative it may be described as a "working diagnosis". This means that other possible diagnoses are still being considered. "Rule out" is a phrase often used by doctors to indicate which of other possible diagnosis are believed to be not as likely.

Diagnosis of the condition is important for proper treatment. For example the symptom of being unable to concentrate and perform well in school has many benign causes, but could also be the result of any one of several different disorders — depression, anxiety, attention deficit disorder, or schizophrenia. Each of these diagnosis is best treated by a different type of medication. The wrong medication will not help and, indeed may make matters worse. It is true, however, that in a few instances the treatment of separate and distinct conditions may share a helpful medication component. For example, the medication Prozac has been effectively used as part of the treatment for depression, obsessive compulsive, and panic disorders.

Child psychiatrists know the various disorders, know the different stages of children's development, and have working clinical experience with the effects of medication. When research is insufficient to provide a clear scientific basis for decision making their expertise and clinic judgement become paramount.

Additional questions for the doctor that parents have found helpful;

- Is the medication called by any other name?

- What is it used for?

- Is it used for anything other than what it is being used for in my child?

- Are there other medications you could use instead?

- Why did you recommend this one?
- Are there side effects that can affect my child's school performance?
- What side effects could occur that you would need to know about?
- When should you be called immediately, or wait until your office opens?
- Are there other medications or foods my child should know to avoid while taking this medication?
- Are there any activities my child should avoid while taking this medication?
- How long do you feel my child may need this medication?
- How will we know if the medication is working?
- How long might that take?
- Will any tests or other blood work have to be done before or during the course of medication?
- How often and where?
- When and how should I give the medication?
- What happens if we miss a dose?
- What happens if the medicine is abruptly stopped?
- Can my child become addicted to this medication?
- Do you have any written information on this drug?
- What is the cost of the medication?
- How will this be written into my child's treatment plan and shared with others on the care team, including those at school?

1. Medication in children and Youth with Emotional, Behavioral-and-Mental Health needs, Florida Dept of Children and Families June 2003, P. 25

Chapter 4

General Advice About Medication

~~~

Everyone for whom medication is prescribed should have a general physical examination. Underlying medical conditions, past medical history, allergies, use of herbal supplements and vitamins, use of medications prescribed by other doctors, use of street drugs or alcohol, and any possibility of pregnancy must all be known to the doctors so that they are able to make good decisions about the use, or choice of medication.

Medications should be used just as the doctor has directed. Discuss beforehand what to do if a dose is missed, or abruptly stopped.

When a medication seems "not to be working" several questions need to be answered:

1.) Has the prescription been filled correctly?

2.) Has the child remembered to take the medication?

3.) Has the medication been taken at the prescribed time?

4.) Has the medication actually been swallowed rather than hidden in the cheek to be spit out later?

If there is no ready explanation for the apparent lack of response DO NOT STOP or INCREASE the dosage on your own. CALL THE DOCTOR.

Subsequent discussions with the doctor may need to address additional questions:

1.) Can the effect of the medication be increased by prescribing a larger dose?

2.) Has sufficient time been allowed for the medication to have a therapeutic effect?

3.) When should a change in medication be considered?

4.) When does the lack of response to "appropriate" medication raise doubt about the accuracy of the diagnosis being treated?

Any medication can cause an allergic reaction. Rashes, itching, and hives are common skin reactions. More serious reactions can cause tissues to swell resulting in problems in the joints, in the digestive tract, or in breathing. Taking more than one medication at a time, may cause increased side effects, and may decrease the desired beneficial effect. Always get advice from your doctor or pharmacist before adding any prescribed, or OVER-THE-COUNTER medication.

Brand name and generic medications may differ in their ingredients and could have some different effects. Color may be different with different dyes causing possible allergic reactions.

Inert fillers or binders may affect the rate of drug release and absorption with possible variations in effect. Always obtain your doctor's advice as to whether a brand name prescription should be used or if a generic medication may be substituted. In the State of New Jersey if a physician has not indicated a preference, your pharmacist is required to offer you the less expensive generic when available.

Chapter 5

Parent Doctor Relationship

Obtaining optimal benefit from medication is achieved by parents and doctors working together. A parent-professional partnership results in a more effective therapeutic alliance. To communicate effectively and build this relationship parents should know:

1.) How to learn more about the child's illness.

2.) The child's complete medical history.

3.) How to maintain a meaningful written record of all medication used (past and present) See p. 16 Medication Log

4.) How the drugs work.

5.) Size and frequency of doses.

6.) Desired effect of medication.

7.) What are the clear indicators of desired effect that need to be observed and tracked.

8.) Side-effects frequency.

9.) Undesired side-effects.

10.) What are the possible serious dangers of the prescribed medications?

11.) How, why, and when to communicate with the doctor directly.

12.) How to contact other involved professionals.

Medication Log

Start Date	Name of Medication	Reason for Use	Mg Daily Dose am/am/pm/pm	Beneficial Effects	Side Effects	Stop Date	Reason for Stopping General Comments
example 1-10-04	Ritalin	poor concentration distractability	10/10/5	better grades	slight weight loss 1st month	8-8-05	stopped for allergic skin rash had good effect on concentration

Chapter 6

What Should Parents Do?

Having a child with an emotional or behavioral disorder affects the entire household and changes the whole pattern of family functioning. Trying to understand what is happening, what can be done, and how to get what the child needs, become overwhelming preoccupations. A growing feeling of self-doubt, accompanied by a barrage of professional directions combine to create a sense of having lost both any control over the situation and the capacity for self-direction. But remember parents and caregivers are the most effective therapeutic agent and need to still be in charge. They need to continue what they do best. They need to continue to parent and promote:

1) **A supportive; safe environment**
   Continuing to be there and staying in touch is the most important support; tolerating that which cannot be immediately changed, or controlled prevents further escalation and helps diffuse and even out crisis.

2) **A regular schedule**
   Routine and predictability are very reassuring to children and reduces their stress and anxiety.

3) **Regular and sufficient sleep**
   Sleep is needed for a sense of well being and optimal function; helps avoid increased irritability and emotional lability caused by fatigue.

4) **Regular exercise**
   Physical activity maintains physical health as well as increasing a sense of well being. Numerous studies have proved exercise to be very effective in reducing both depression and anxiety.

5) **Regular and nutritious meals**
   Diet should avoid simple sugars. A diet with sweets will produce sugar "highs" and cause troublesome over-activity. Sugar "highs" are followed by "lows" which cause anxiety, irritability, and weakness. Carbohydrates are an important part of the diet should be of the complex variety that are digested slowly and provide a continued steady source of energy. Artificial "foods", additives, and stimulants should be avoided.

6) **Good physical health**
   The signs and symptoms of **physical** illness can be masked and overlooked in the midst of other problems. Periodic physical exams are important.

7) **Good brain health**
   TV has become the biggest purveyor of what is fed into children's brains. Active involvement and creativity in determining a child's TV diet produces good food for thought, and better brain health. Remember all children under 3 are unable to differentiate make believe from reality. Early TV exposure to violence can lead to its acceptance as part of normal behavior free from consequences.

   Personal computers should be avoided in early childhood, and later their use needs supervision. The pop culture of introducing children to personal computers as early as possible can be problematic to the development of many "normal" children, and can be a serious pitfall for some children with emotional problems. Before children have the capacity for critical reasoning children "check out" the meaning of words by "reading" the facial expression of the speaker. Computers by-pass this early, innate critical ability. Unknowingly the child can be led into a fantasy world cloaked with a few appearances of reality. The enjoyable interaction process, free from the stress of real human interaction and reinforced by electronic rewards, can become a preferred activity for children. Those with an anxious temperament are even more vulnerable.

Do not forget that as parents or caregivers you HAVE to look after yourself. Start by determining the limits of your own physical and mental strength. Decide what you can do, and identify what you cannot. By clarifying your capabilities you can be more focused on what specific help you need. Identifying needs is the first step in getting them met.

Support groups are a valuable resource and can make a critical difference. To know that you and your family are not alone and to know others have survived is of great help. Groups provide education and practical "know how", for example, how other parents have handled similar problems. In sharing your experience, your pain, and what you have learned, strong, mutually supportive relationships develop.

To find a NAMI support group in New Jersey call (732) 940-0991
(For all other states see pp. 107-113)

Chapter 7

How Medications Work

The nerve cell **(neuron)** is the basic working unit of the nervous system and functions to conduct electrical stimuli to other cells. It can receive multiple input messages through its numerous **dendrites** and send an electric message through its single **axon.**

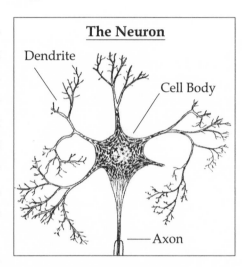

The Neuron

Dendrite

Cell Body

Axon

The neuron is a small electrical conducting system which has multiple specialized areas on its surface that control its activity. These areas are called **receptors** and can signal the neuron to "go" or to "stop".

All drugs prescribed for emotional and behavioral disorders act directly upon the neuron to produce one of the three following effects:

1.) Affect the "go" ● receptor to **turn on** the the neuron and create electrical activity. These drugs are called ACTIVATORS. Some of these medications are also called stimulants.

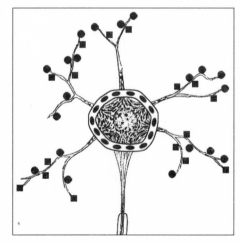

2.) Affect the "stop" ■ receptor to **turn off,** the neuron by inhibiting electrical activity. These drugs are called INHIBITORS.

3.) Affect "caution" ⬭ and restraint by making it difficult for the neuron to conduct electrical activity along its surface **(membrane).** Drugs that decrease the spread of activity to surrounding neurons have a stabilizing effect. Because these drugs were first used to prevent convulsions they were called anticonvulsants. Today these medications are also referred to as mood STABILIZERS.

The relatively simple drug effects **(turn on, turn off, or stabilize)** can bring about changes in complex human behavior by altering the strength of connections between neurons or neuron groups. Just as a train can be routed by throwing a railroad switch, so too can the direction and destination of a train of thought be determined by increasing the (synaptic) strength of neuronal connections and thereby create a preferred track among a myriad of alternatives.

Chapter 8

Structure and Function
of the Brain

~~~⌒

The basic function of the brain is to receive information (in the form of sensory perceptions), recognize the pattern of this incoming information from previous experience and then make an appropriate response.

There are approximately 100 billion neurons in the brain. Of these only 2.5 million neurons are used to receive information and only 1.25 million to make a response. This leaves over 99% of the brain cells to hold the new experience in working memory, search through stores of previous similar experience, "think" of all possible courses of action, and then choose the best response. Only part of this analysis and thinking is done in the realm of conscious awareness.

The cerebral cortex has 28 billion neurons. Different groups of these neurons have developed highly specialized skills in separate parts of the brain (LOBES). (Figure 1).

Cerebral Mapping

While the lobes of the cerebral cortex are endowed with a basic form, their ultimate structure is completed only by responding to environmental influences. Each type of stimulus is routed to an appropriate lobe—i.e. what is seen by the eye is conducted to the visual cortex in the occipital lobe for further processing. Each lobe of the cerebral cortex contains sheets of loosely connected neurons called maps where learned information is stored.

The synapse with its special variability provides a biologic mechanism which allows the brain to self-organize and learn on

Lobes of the Cerebral Cortex and Their Specialized Functions

Figure 1

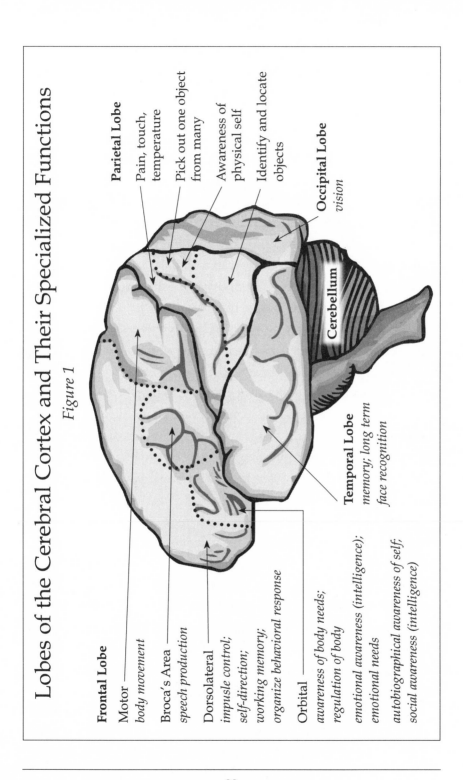

Frontal Lobe

Motor
body movement

Broca's Area
speech production

Dorsolateral
*impulse control;
self-direction;
working memory;
organize behavioral response*

Orbital
*awareness of body needs;
regulation of body*

*emotional awareness (intelligence);
emotional needs*

*autobiographical awareness of self;
social awareness (intelligence)*

Parietal Lobe

Pain, touch, temperature

Pick out one object from many

Awareness of physical self

Identify and locate objects

Occipital Lobe
vision

Cerebellum

Temporal Lobe
*memory; long term
face recognition*

its own. A new perception when conducted to the sensory specific area (neuronal map), will cause a number of random neurons to be activated at the same instant. Simultaneous activation and firing cause their neuronal interconnections (SYNAPSES) to grow stronger. A synapse is similar to a muscle in that the more it is used the stronger it becomes. Thus an original random group of neurons develops strengthened synapses and starts to function as a specific unit each time the "new" experience is subsequently encountered. This unit of neurons, connected to fire simultaneously, are said to form a neuronal representation, or neuronal image, of that experience. Here "image" does not refer to a visual perception but rather to the creation of a representation by a specific group of neurons. With the formation of an image the experience is "learned" and, if significant, its image will be engraved in long term memory. These remembered images of past experience are pieces of meaning which we use to construct our experience of the present.

Take for example a doughnut. Our visual map has an image of a "ring shape", our tactile sensory map contributes a representation of "soft and sticky", while a taste map adds an image of "sweetness", and smell map a "fresh doughiness". All of these images mapped in separate lobes of the brain are then simultaneously and seamlessly integrated into a moment of eating a doughnut.

In the brain images of objects with very similar characteristics are stored in the same area. Thus a representation of doughnut, cookie, and cake are clustered on the same neuronal map.

The brain can extend this same process to make a map of other maps which share a meaningful characteristic. For example the doughnut-cookie-cake map could be grouped by commonality on a map which already holds a corn-rice-potato map.

The ability to group objects and "finding" the common characteristic is the neurologic mechanism creating abstract thinking

The frontal lobe has the greatest capacity for progressive hierarchial classification. (Figure 2).

Mapping in the Lobes of the Cerebral Cortex

Figure 2

Level of Map	Subject of Mapping	Location	Function of Mapping Common characteristic / Result
1	Ring shape, sticky, sweet	All sensory lobes	Recognition of Object Result: Doughnut
2	Doughnut, cookies, cake	Parietal	Grouping of Objects Result: Carbohydrate
3	Carbohydrates, protein, fat	Parietal Frontal	Classification of Groupings Result: Food
4	Food, shelter, clothing	Frontal	Abstraction of Classifications Result: Necessities
5	Etcetera	Frontal	

The Synapse

A synapse is the structure formed where the end (TERMINAL) of a neuron sending a message is very close to a specialized area of the receiving neuron (DENDRITIC SPINE) (Figure 3). The sending neuron's terminal releases a chemical messenger (NEUROTRANSMITTER), which moves across a small gap to fit into a specific receptor on the receiving dendritic spine. At the receptor a series of chemical reactions takes place which activates the neuron to generate an electric current down its axon to complete the transmission. (Figure 4)

Direct connection of one neuron to another would insure the electric message is rapidly transmitted without any interruption or delay. Why is there a gap between neurons that requires bridging by such a complicated system of neurotransmitters and neuroreceptors?

A neuron has the capacity to be connected to anywhere from 4,000 to 10,000 other neurons. A neuron could receive literally thousands of incoming influences—some stimulating and some inhibiting. Thus a single neuron can "decide" whether to act by adding up the positive and negative inputs. The synaptic structure also provides a mechanism whereby an impulse can be greatly amplified by releasing a large amount of neurotransmitter. Another advantage is that nerve transmission can be halted by a synapse whereas direct connection would be unfailingly conducted. But perhaps the greatest advantage of the synapse structure is that it allows the connection between neurons to be changeable, to be plastic, and thus to be adaptable to new experience. This plasticity stems from the remarkable ability of each of our brain's neurons to vary the number of axon terminals, the number of receptors, the rate of neurotransmitter production, the rate of carrying away neurotransmitters by re-uptake transporter proteins, and by the rate of enzymatic breakdown.

The process of learning is the process of making connections between different concepts or perceptions. The variable and plastic synapse enables new connections to be made with new experiences. This allows us to learn and to be able to adapt to new environments.

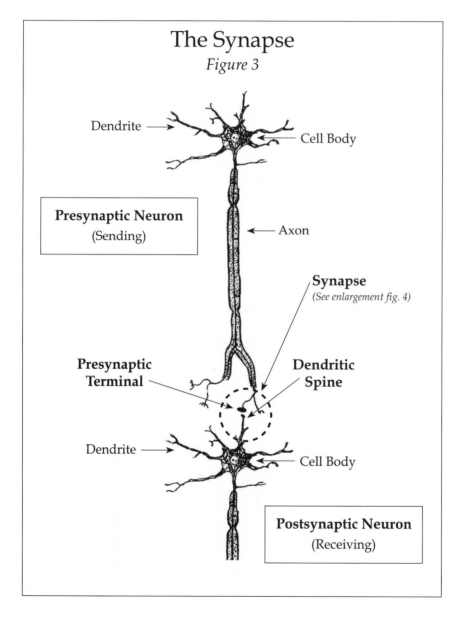

The Synapse
Figure 3

Dendrite

Cell Body

Presynaptic Neuron
(Sending)

Axon

Synapse
(See enlargement fig. 4)

Presynaptic Terminal

Dendritic Spine

Dendrite

Cell Body

Postsynaptic Neuron
(Receiving)

The Synapse

Figure 4

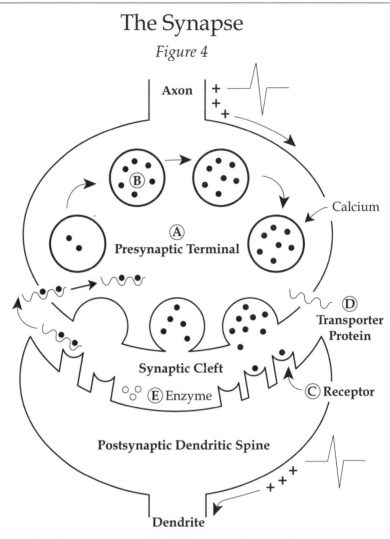

Strength of synaptic connection can be changed by varying:

(A) The number of presynaptic terminals

(B) The rate of neurotransmitter production

(C) The number of receptors

(D) Removal of neurotransmitter by re-uptake transporters

(E) Enzymatic destruction of neurotransmitter

Evolution of the Brain

Figure 5

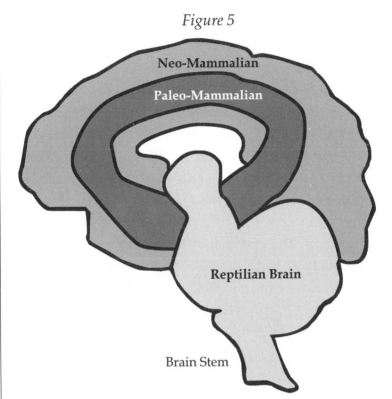

The brain has evolved thru three major developmental stages.

- [ ] The first stage is reptilian and contains the brain stem where all basic life functions are supported. Deep within its center lie the origins of the neuromodulators.

- [x] The second stage PALEO-MAMMALIAN denotes the evolution of mammals with maternal instincts and a complex system of emotional communication between mother and off-spring

- [ ] The third stage NEO-MAMMALIAN is characterized by marked growth of the cerebral cortex, particularly in the region of the frontal lobes which house speech production and increased complexity of thinking.

Neurotransmitters

Different types of chemical substances have the ability to bridge the gap (SYNAPTIC CLEFT) separating neurons. Amino acids, amines, small pieces of protein (PEPTIDES) and even some gases have been found to have this capacity.

The cerebral cortex (NEOCORTEX) is the most recent part of the brain to develop and use the "modern" neurotransmitters. Twenty eight billion cells in the cerebral cortex use the new amino acid transmitters. These neurotransmitters are very fast and respond in millionths of a second. They act in a very small local area and are very specific and precise. They also are relatively efficient in that they are easily regenerated from food sources and never wear out or become exhausted. These neurotransmitters actively participate in the perception, storage, and analysis of information. But since they do not play a primary role in emotional and behavioral disorders they are beyond the scope of this discussion. The single exception is GABA (gamma amino butyric acid) which plays a universal role of inhibition in all parts of the brain.

Neuromodulators

The neurons whose neurotransmitters serve to control and regulate other neurons are called neuromodulators. These neuromodulators originate in the oldest part of the brain, the brain stem, and are quite different from the "new" neurotransmitters in the cerebral cortex. The concept of "old" and "new" refers to the three evolutionary stages of brain development. (Figure 5)

In the "new" part of the brain, neourotransmitters can react in millionths of a second, when someone is, for example, performing mathematical calculations. However neurotransmitters which regulate emotion and feeling are fortunately much slower.

Serotonin, dopamine and norepinephrine are three neuromodulators that reach out from the old brain stem to regulate and integrate the newer more highly specialized cerebral cortex. (Fig. 6). Thus even complex thinking cannot be totally free from influences stemming from that part of the brain concerned with sustaining life.

Neuromodulators not only create a system whereby brain activity is coordinated and regulated, but they also initiate adaptive changes in the brain itself. Neuromodulators act upon G-protein receptors of neurons. These G-protein receptors bring about a whole cascade of chemical reactions. Each chemical reaction effects the function of the nerve cell. At the very end of the cascade, chemical signals are produced to turn genes on or off. These genes then manufacture proteins that physically alter the nerve cells. These alterations of nerve cells, in turn, modify the activity of the individual. Thus stimuli originating in the environment can bring about adaptive changes both in physical structure and behavior.

Important Neuromodulators

Figure 6

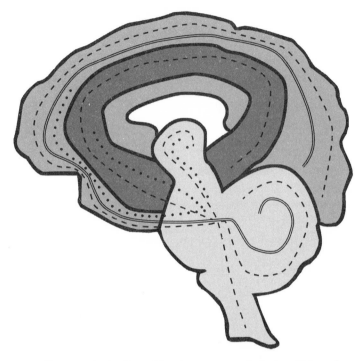

- - - - Serotonin is the oldest neuromodulator. It has been identified in organisms which existed 800,000,000 years ago. It's wide spread distribution explains the great clinical diversity of serotonin effects.

• • • • • • With the evolution of brains the addition of dopamine provided a basis for instinctual drives, and other "feel good" experiences as well as the more subtle forms of motivation that underlie curiosity and the inner rewards of learning.

═══ Norepinephrine is the most recent neuromodulator. It is distributed in the newest cerebral cortex where it enhances alertness, selects "important" stimuli, and then appropriately focus brain activity.

Chapter 9

Classification of Drugs

Psychoactive medications have been classified by several different criteria—i.e. chemical characteristics, clinical use, or mechanism of action. A new approach is used here which is simpler and more practical. New knowledge of the specialized function of different parts of the brain provides the needed and logical connection between drug action and behavioral change.

This approach provides a mental framework to organize information about drugs. Not only does this provide a better understanding of medications effects but provides an opportunity for participation in the process of drug selection. Knowledge that serotonin can have a beneficial effect on depression, further suggests all drugs with a strong serotonin effect could be considered as possible therapeutic choices. This approach can be helpful in establishing better communication with the doctor.

All psychoactive drugs have one of three basic functions—activate, inhibit, or stabilize. The activators group has the largest number of effective drugs. Any drugs can be said to have a psychopharmacological effect only in as much as they have an effect on one or more of the neuromodulators systems—norepinephrine, dopamine, and serotonin.

Increasing numbers of people with mental illness have been found to have variations in their receptors for neuromodulators and other parts of the brain. The discovery of alterations in the physical structure of the brain has worked to redefine "mental illness". Mental illness is now seen as a biological disease of the brain which can produce changes in thinking, emotions and behavior.

Activating medications will now be discussed as to how they influence these three neuromodulator systems.

Chapter 10

Types of Medication

Activators

Norepinephrine System

Dopamine System

Serotonin System

Norepinephrine System

There are only 50,000 neurons in the norepinephrine system. They originate in the part of the brain stem called the locus ceruleus. By means of synapses using norepinephrine as the neurotransmitter, these cells perform important alerting functions in the posterior parietal lobe and the anterior frontal lobe.

In the attentional system located in the right parietal lobe norepinephrine functions like a TV's "contrast knob" by increasing incoming signal from background noise. Signals identifying important objects are intensified and stand out from the general input from the outside world. This important information is then sent to the frontal lobe. Here norepinephrine cells activate the frontal attention system, which uses its own separate dopamine transmitter to decrease general activity, suppress impulsive reactions, and allow time to think about the most appropriate response.

Norepinephrine is also involved with a fear and arousal mechanism. When there is increased activity of the locus ceruleus, excessive norepinephrine stimulation of the amygdala (the center for conditioned fear) may lead to the development of post-trau-matic stress disorder.

Some medications with a norepinephrine effect mixed with either a serotonin, or dopamine effect, have also been found to be effective in the treatment of depression.

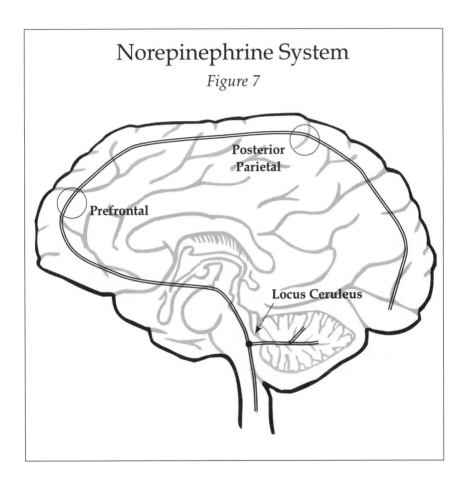

Norepinephrine System
Figure 7

Normal Levels of Norepinephrine

Function:	Associated Activity:
regulate arousal	attention
provides alerting	memory
directs attention to behaviorally signification stimuli	learning adaptation
regulates internal self in accordance to outside world	socialization
stimulates sympathetic nervous system	Fight or flight response
stimulates dopamine system in Prefrontal cortex	control impulse inhibition

Low Levels of Norepinephrine

Function:	Associated Activity:
decrease signal/noise from posterior parietal cortex decrease orientation to new stimuli decrease attention to new stimuli	attention deficit disorder
decrease signal/noise from prefrontal cortex decrease attention attention decrease in inhibitory control	deficit hyperactivity disorder

High Levels of Norepinephrine

Function:	Associated Activity:
over arousal	anxiety disorder
over stimulation of sympathetic nervous system (pounding heart, tremor)	panic attack
impairment of internal regulation of self	post-traumatic stress disorder

Norepinephrine (Adrenergic) Receptors

Norepinephrine has two basic types of receptors, alpha and beta, which tend to balance each other's separate and opposing functions. Differences in alpha receptors are indicated by alpha 1 and alpha 2. Alpha 1 receptors are only on the receiving postsynaptic side of the synapse. Alpha 2 receptors are primarily distributed on the sending pre-synaptic side. (Figure 8).

The postsynaptic neuron is stimulated when its alpha 1 adrenergic receptor is activated by norepinephrine.

When a norepinephrine neuron has produced sufficient neurotransmitter, excess amounts reach the presynaptic alpha 2 adrenergic receptor, which then curtails norepinephrine release. This auto-receptor provides a self-regulating capability.

Norepinephrine Neuron with Adrenergic Receptors

Presynaptic Alpha 2 and Post-synaptic Alpha 1

Figure 8

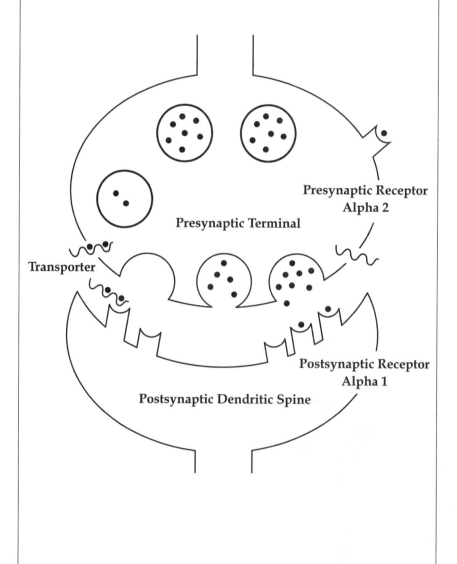

Presynaptic Receptor
Alpha 2

Presynaptic Terminal

Transporter

Postsynaptic Receptor
Alpha 1

Postsynaptic Dendritic Spine

Alpha Stimulators
Catapres (clonidine) and Tenex (guanfacine)

Description

Catapres and Tenex are two medications that have been approved for use in the treatment of high blood pressure. They have a norepinephrine effect when acting upon alpha 2 receptors and are called "alpha 2 adrenergic agonists".

Mechanism of Action

Both medications preferentially activate presynaptic alpha 2 receptors and reduce norepinephrine effects of brain excitation, increased motor activity, and increased environmental input from the posterior attentional system. As a result, these medications have a quieting, calming or even sedating effect.

Some activation of the post-synaptic alpha 2 receptor turns on the anterior attentional system in the frontal lobe which decreases motor activity, inhibits impulsive reactions, and generates thoughtful responses.

Indicators and Uses

These medications are used for attention deficit hyperactivity disorders particularly when there is extreme hyperactivity, low frustration threshold and emotional outbursts. Use of these medications has been effective in the treatment of oppositional disorder, conduct disorder, aggressive behavior, self-injury behavior, agitation, anxiety and insomnia. When use in Tourette's syndrome impulsivity and hyperactivity have been reduced.

Tenex, when compared to Catapres, has a longer duration of action, less sedation, and more effectiveness for inattention.

Side Effects

Sedation is most common early in treatment but tends to improve after several weeks. Dry mouth; slower heart rate; loss of appetite; nausea; vomiting; weakness; nervousness; skin rash; less frequent agitation and depression.

Monitoring

Because electrical conduction in the heart can be slowed, it is advisable to have an electrocardiogram before starting on the medications.

Blood pressure and pulse rate need to be checked periodically to detect the possibility of excessive lowering.

Warnings

MEDICATION SHOULD NOT BE STOPPED ABRUPTLY because a serious withdrawal problem could result. Sudden removal of a suppressing effect could be followed by a period of abrupt over activity. This "rebound" effect could result in nervousness, agitation, insomnia, headache, high blood pressure and rapid heart rate. BE CAREFUL NOT TO LET PRESCRIPTIONS RUN OUT.

What Else You Need to Know

The word "Clonidine" can be easily misheard and confused with Klonopin. Always double check the labels when picking up prescriptions.

Soaking of the patch system can change the amount of Catapress released and absorbed. A child should not swim with a Catapress skin patch. Rather is should be removed, and after swimming replace with a new patch. Protective covers are supplied for showering.

Strattera (atomoxetine)

Description

This is a new non-stimulant medication that increases norepinephrine and has been proven to be safe in children 6 years of age and older.

Mechanism of Action

Interferes with the transporter re-uptake system for norepinphrine in the presynaptic neuron.

Stimulates dopamine in prefrontal cortex.

Indications and Uses

It is used in the treatment of attention deficit and attention deficit hyperactivity disorders.

Side Effects

The most common side effects are upset stomach, decreased appetite, nausea or vomiting. Less frequently; dizziness, tiredness, mood swings. In young adults additional side effects may include difficulty in urinating, menstrual cramps, or sexual problems.

Monitoring

Blood pressure and pulse should be checked to detect any undesired increases or decreases in blood pressure and pulse.

Warnings

- Do not use within two weeks of taking any monoamine oxidase inhibitors.
- Can cause mania in bipolar disorder.
- Rarely can cause severe liver damage (recent warning).

What Else You Need to Know

If child loses weight or fails to gain weight normally, notify your doctor. Angioneurotic edema is an allergic reaction that has occurred uncommonly.

Norepinephrine System Drugs

Drug	Units in MGs	Usual Daily Dose MGs	Duration of Effect	Ususal # Doses/Day	Rate of Dose Change
Catapres (clonidine)	.1, .2, .3	.15–30	4–6 hours	3–4 times	.05 mgs/3days
Tenex (guanfacine)	1, 2	1–3.0	6–8 hours	2 times	.5 mgs/3days
Strattera (atomoxetine)	10, 18, 25	40–100	5–24 hours	1–2 times	40 mgs/week
(reboxetine) (Not in the U.S. yet)	2 mgm	2–4 (max 6)		1–2 times	

Norepinephrine System Drugs

Drug	Advantages	Disadvantages	Norepinephrine Effect	Dopamine Effect	Serotonin Effect
Catapres (clonidine)	Most helpful with extreme over activity, aggression, conduct disorder, self-injury, agitation	Less effective for pure inattention, stop gradually, sedation, dry mouth, dizziness rare: agitation	++++	+	0
Tenex (guanfacine)	same	same	++++	+	0
Strattera (atomoxetine)	no sedation fewer side effects	dry mouth, nausea, constipation	++++	++	0
(reboxetine) (Not in the U.S. yet)	few side effects	same–milder	++++	(prefrontal) 0	0

BETA Blockers
Corgard (nadolol), Inderal (propranolol), Tenormin (atenolol), Visken (pindolol).

Description

Beta blockers are a class of medication that have been used in the treatment of heart disease, high blood pressure and heart beat irregularities. Some of the more common members of this class included:

Corgard (nadolol)   Tenormin (atenolol)

Inderal (propranolol)   Visken (pindolol)

Mechanism of Action

Tenormin (atenolol) blocks B1, adrenergic receptors selectively while the others block both B1 and B2. By blocking adrenergic receptors neuron activity is inhibited and reduced.

Indications and Uses

These medications are very effective in reducing the troubling symptoms of anxiety such as tremor, shakiness, sweating, feeling of over-stimulation with rapid heart-beat and pulse. They are of benefit in reducing excitement, agitation, and aggression. Single doses are sometimes used to reduce performance anxiety (stage fright).

Side Effects

Side effects are generally more troublesome with higher doses and include tingling and numbness of fingers, tiredness, weakness, low blood pressure slow heart beat, dizziness when standing up quickly. Rarely diarrhea, insomnia, nightmares, muscle cramps.

Monitoring

Pulse and standing blood pressure should be monitored, particularly when first starting the medication.

Warnings

Can precipitate severe wheezing if asthma is present. Medication should be discontinued gradually to prevent withdrawal rebound of emotional disturbance, rapid heart beat, and rise in blood pressure.

What Else You Should Know

- Can cause depression and short term memory loss.

- Can cause hallucinations.

- Can block the warning symptoms of low blood sugar in individuals with diabetes.

BETA–Blockers

Drug	How Supplied MG	Usual Daily MG in 24 hrs	Ususal # Doses/Day
Corgard (nadolol)	20, 40, 80	10–80	1
Inderal (propranolol)	10, 20, 40, 60, 80	10–100	2
Tenormin (atenolol)	25, 50, 100	12.5–100	1
Visken (pindolol)	5, 10	2.5–10	1

Dopamine System

Dopamine evolved with the development of the brain. The dopamine system is comprised of only 250,000 neurons originating in three areas of the brain. While participating in the earliest stages of fetal brain formation, full development takes almost 20 years.

Dopamine is most active in the anticipation of possible rewards and provides incentives for behavior. It's motivating effects activate the attention system, enhance working memory, and cognitive planning efforts. The motor system is primed and prepared to move quickly towards the targeted goal.

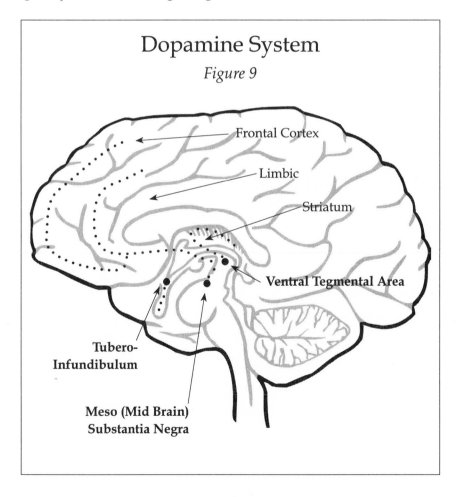

Dopamine System

Figure 9

Frontal Cortex

Limbic

Striatum

Ventral Tegmental Area

Tubero-Infundibulum

Meso (Mid Brain)
Substantia Negra

Dopamine drives physical appetites as well as providing rewards for mental accomplishments such as learning. It is dopamine that provides the highs of cocaine use, and it is changes in the dopamine system that result in addiction.

Diseases that diminish dopamine, such as Parkinson's Disease, result in decreased motor activity, emotional activity, and cognitive ability. High levels of dopamine result in increased motor activity, stimulus seeking behavior, and aggression. Excessive dopamine secretion in the limbic system can cause disturbances of perception and result in psychosis.

The dopamine system plays an important role in Attention Deficit Hyperactivity Disorder (ADHD) as well as schizophrenia.

Role of Dopamine in ADHD

As our understanding increases, we will come to appreciate many different ways a child's brain can be affected to produce a common behavior we identify as ADHD.

In the resting state the rate of dopamine release by neurons is constant for any given child. This results in an even baseline level of dopamine released into the synaptic space. The dopamine secreting neurons have a self-regulating turn off mechanism (auto-receptor) to prevent excessive dopamine release. This mechanism requires an adequate maintenance level of dopamine to prime it and have it function smoothly. In ADHD the baseline level of dopamine is well below the normal baseline. When a child with ADHD experiences an exciting event, with subsequent increases in the release of dopamine the turn off mechanism is delayed. The dopamine, release is too prolonged and becomes "out of control".

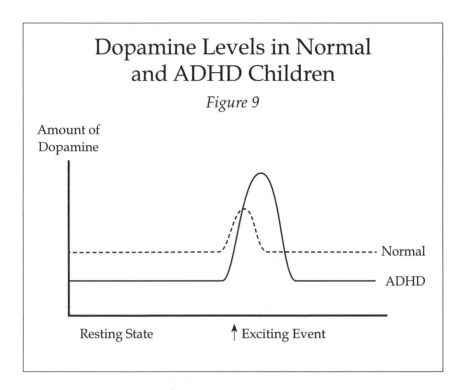

Dopamine Levels in Normal and ADHD Children

Figure 9

- Treatment of ADHD with dopamine stimulators raises the resting dopamine level and enhances the self-regulating system to control excessive dopamine release.

- Dopamine facilitates the anterior attention system in the left frontal lobe.

- Dopamine activates the inhibition center in the right frontal lobe.

Dopamine Stimulators
Ritalin, Metadate, Concerta,
Focalin (methylphenidate)

Description

Methylphenidate is a mild brain stimulant. The four brands above differ in the mechanism of, rate of and predictability of drug release. Focalin is a dextro isomer and is fast acting and has twice the potency of all other forms of methyphenidate. Ritalin is fast acting but is also available in a sustained release (SR) form. Metadate extended release (ER) provides a more reliable form of once a day dosing. Concerta combines an outer immediate release layer with an inner osmotic pump mechanism which gives very reliable steady drug release.

Mechanism of Action

Methylphenidate acts by increasing the amount of dopamine in the synaptic space. This is achieved by inhibition of the transporter system for dopamine re-uptake by the presynaptic neuron.

Indications and Uses

Primary indication is for ADHD. It is also approved for use in narcolepsy.

Side Effects

Nervousness and insomnia are most common and may be controlled by adjusting dosage; allergic skin rash, dizziness; headache; abdominal pain; changes in blood pressure and pulse.

Monitoring

Liver function tests at discretion of physician.

Warnings

Should not be used in epilepsy as seizure threshold is reduced. Can produce motor tics and be problematic in Tourette's syndrome. Severe nervousness and thought disorders can be aggravated.

What Else You Should Know

- Can produce dependence in addictive personality.

- Decrease in appetite is not infrequent

- Decrease in rate of growth is possible, but reversible with discontinuing medication

- Has become the most popular drug on college campuses because of enhanced attention and concentration even in "normal" students.

Dopamine Stimulators
Dexedrine (dextroamphetamine)
Adderall (amphetamine) and Cylert (pemoline)

Description

Dexedrine is the d-isomer of amphetamine, Adderall is the mixture of four different amphetamine salts. Cylert is chemically unrelated but is included because of its identical mild brain stimulation effects.

Mechanism of Action

All three drugs act by increasing dopamine in the synaptic space. Amphetamine effects are complex in that it stimulates dopamine release, inhibits re-uptake removal, and reduces enzymatic breakdown.

Indications and Uses

Primary indication is for ADHD. Amphetamines are also approved for use in narcolepsy.

Side Effects

Nervousness and insomnia most common, allergic, skin rash, dizziness, headache, abdominal pain, changes in pulse and blood pressure.

Monitoring

Reports of cylert causing life threatening liver failure requires regular liver function tests.

Warnings

- Cylert has caused FATAL LIVER DAMAGE in rare instances

- Should not be used in epilepsy as seizures threshold is reduced.

- Can produce motor tics and be problematic in Tourette's syndrome

- Severe nervousness and thought disorders can be aggravated.

What Else You Need to Know

Amphetamines are potentially addictive and have an extensive history of abuse. However, keep in mind a child with ADHD well controlled with prescribed medication, has a much lower risk of developing substance abuse, as compared to a child whose ADHD is not treated, and not controlled.

Dopamine System Drugs (Stimulators)

Drug	Units in MGs	Usual Daily Dose MGs	Duration of Effect	Ususal # Doses/Day	Rate of Dose Change
Ritalin (methylphenidate)	5, 10, 20SR	2.5 BID–15 TID .5 BID–20 TID 10 BID–20 TID	2–4 hours SR 6 hours	2–3 times	5–10 per week
Focalin (methylphinidate)	2.5, 5, 10	2.5–10 BID	2–4 hours	2 times	2.5–5 per week
Dexedrine (dextroamphetamine)	5, 10, 15	1.2 BID–7.5 TID 2.5 BID–10 TID 5 BID–10 TID	3–5 hours	2–3 times	5 per week
Adderall (4 salt mixture of amphetamine)	5, 10, 15	Same	3–5 hours	1–2 times	5 per week
Cylert (pemoline)	18.7, 37.5, 75	37.5–112.5	12–24 hours	1 time	after 3–4 weeks 18.7 per week
Concerta (methylphenidate)	18, 36, 54	18 QAM	12 hours	1 time	18 per week
Metadate (methylphenidate)	10, 20		12 hours	1 time	10 per week

Dopamine System Drugs (Stimulators)

Drug	Advantages	Disadvantages	Norepinephrine Effect	Dopamine Effect	Serotonin Effect
Ritalin (methylphenidate)	few negative effects	too short acting	+	++++	0
Focalin (methylphinidate)	few negative effects	too short acting	+	++++	0
Dexedrine (dextroamphetamine)	longer acting	labeled "speed" high abuse potential decreased growth	++	++++	+
Adderall (amphetamine) (dextroamphetamine)	reliable can use > 3YO	abuse potential decreased growth	++	++++	+
Cylert (pemoline)	not labeled	slow 3–4 weeks not approved < 6YO under age of 60	0	++++	0
Concerta (methylphenidate)	1 time/day		++	++++	0
Metadate (methylphenidate)	1 time/day		++	++++	0

The Role of Dopamine in Schizophrenia

In the 1950's it was serendipitously discovered that chlorpromazine helped persons with schizophrenia. The drug shared structural similarities with dopamine and fit into but did not activate the receptor. This essentially blocked the dopamine D2 receptor. The dopamine blocker medications are called neuroleptics.

There are three major dopamine pathways (figure 11). Two of these pathways play a prominent role in Weinberg's dopamine theory of schizophrenia. The mesocortical dopamine pathway is underactive and produces the "negative" symptoms: lack of motivation, lack of planning, lack of spontaneity, inpaired thinking and confusion. The frontal cortex controls the lower limbic system. Lack of sufficient dopamine activity in the frontal lobes allows the limbic system to escape control, become over active and produce the overt "positive" symptoms: emotional disturbance, sensory perception problems, and psychosis. Treatment with neuroleptics block dopamine receptors. Preventing stimulation of dopamine receptors in the limbic system, reduces its over activity. As a result positive symptoms are decreased.

The striatum plays an important role in the whole motor system and also shares a rich distribution of D2 receptors. Thus, early neuroleptic (dopamine blocking) medications were typically accompanied by a variety of undesired movement problems. The newer neuroleptics have a greater effect on other dopamine receptors, have weaker D2 blocking with its associated movement problems, and are therefore called "atypical".

The unwanted side-effects of dopamine blockers are a major concern.

Dopamine Pathways

Figure 11

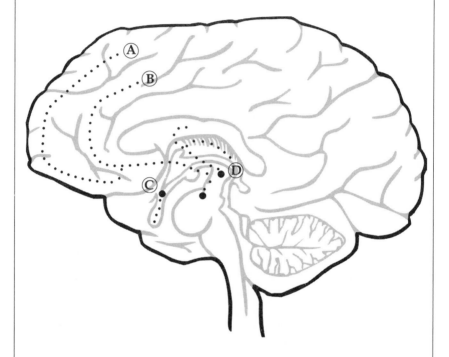

Ⓐ Mesocortical dopamine pathway is involved with attention, motivation, planning, recent memory, thinking, and spontaneous activity.

Ⓑ Mesolimbic dopamine pathway regulates sensory perceptions and emotions.

Ⓒ Tubero-infundibular dopamine pathway controls (inhibits) the secretion of prolactin hormone.

Ⓓ Nigrostriatal dopamine pathway is centrally involved in the brain circuits that regulate movement, emotion, and thinking.

Major Concerns About
Dopamine Blocking Neuroleptics

It is not known if the use of neuroleptics has any effects on the development of the brain.

Blocking dopamine in pathway A (figure 11) can result in decreased attention and memory as well as impaired thinking.

Blocking dopamine in pathway C can increase the secretion of the hormone prolactin which in turn may result in breast development, menstrual irregularity and impaired sexual function.

Blocking dopamine in pathway D can result in any one of several different movement problems:

- **Acute dystonia** (onset hours — days after starting drug) sudden muscular contractions that are involuntary, uncoordinated, and cause distorted movements. Contractions in the head and neck may be more sustained to produce an arching posture, while more often are momentary in the arms and legs to cause jerking.

- **Pseudo-Parkinsonism** (onset 5–30 days) difficulty in initiating and stopping movements, increased muscle tone, slow shuffling walk

- **Akathisia** (Onset 5–60 days) restless discomfort of muscles with inability to remain still and need to move for relief.

- **Tardive dyskinesia** (long term) involuntary writhing movements of face and tongue, rabbit-like quivering with its social disfigurement

Other Side Effects of Neuroleptics

allergic	skin rash
anticholinergic	dryness of mouth and eyes, nasal congestion
brain	drowsiness, sedation rare increase in psychosis, catatonia
endocrine	breast enlargement, menstrual irregularities
gastro-intestinal	constipation, jaundice
metabolic	appetite not turned off, weight gain (exception? Abilify)
cardiovascular	common drop in blood pressure with standing. Electrical changes in heart (prolonged QT interval) possible with Mellaril, Orap, and Geodon. May cause serious changes in heart rhythm.
bone marrow	agranulocytosis (impared ability to manufacture white blood cells) – blood counts needed for Clozaril.

Side Effects
Dopamine System Drugs (Blockers)

Drug Brand	Generic	Sedation	Anticholinergic	Motor
Thorazine	(chlorpromazine)	+++	+++	++
Mellaril	(thioridazine)	+++	+++	+
Trilafon	(perphenazine)	++	+	+++
Stelazine	trifluperazine)	++	+	+
Navane	(triothexene)	+	+	+++
Haldol	(haloperidol)	+	+	+++
Prolixin	(fluphenazine)	+	+	+++
Orap	(pimozide)	+	+	+++
Clozaril	(clozapine)	+++	+++	?0
Risperdal	(risperidone)	++	+	?0
Zyprexa	(olanzapine)	++	+	?0
Seroquel	(quetiapine)	++	++	?0
Geodon	(ziprasidone)	++	++	?+
Abilify	(aripiprazole)	+/-	+	?0
Loxitane	(loxapine)	+	+	+

Anticholinergic side-effects include: dry mouth, visual blurring, constipation, and difficulty in urination.

Neuroleptics

Description

Dopamine blockers are called neuroleptics and are separated into two general groups:

Typical		Atypical	
Thorazine	(chlorpromazine)	Clozaril	(clozapine)
Mellaril	(thioridazine)	Risperdal	(risperidone)
Trilafon	(perphenazine)	Zyprexa	(olanzapine)
Stelazine	(trifluoperazine)	Seroquel	(quetipine)
Navane	(thiothixene)	Geodon	(ziprasidone)
Haldol	(haloperidol)	Abilify	(aripiprazole)
Prolixin	(fluphenazine)		
Orap	(pimozide)		
Loxitane	(loxapine)		

Mechanism of Action

Early neuroleptics strongly blocked the D2 dopamine receptor. The newer atypical neuroleptics have a wider range of dopamine blocking D1 thru D5 with less affinity for D2 receptors and the resulting movement problems.

Indications and Uses

Neuroleptics are used to treat psychosis and schizophrenia, in children with developmental disorders that have attendant stereotypic repetitive movements neuroleptics have been of benefit. Similarly tics may be reduced in Tourette's Syndrome. Other uses include severe aggression, explosive, disorder, and self-injurious behavior. Severe agitation can be controlled and has engendered the term "major tranquilizer" for neuroleptics.

Side Effects
pp. 57-59

Monitoring

Clozaril   weekly white blood cell count

Cylert   regular liver function tests

Geodon
Mellaril   } electrocardiogram to look for QT interval prolongation and the possibility of serious heart
Orap   arrhythmias

Warnings

Very rare but LIFE THREATENING neuroleptic MALIGNANT SYNDROME the sudden onset of muscular rigidity, elevation of body temperature and collapse of the regulation of the circulatory system.

WHAT ELSE YOU NEED TO KNOW

In rare instances neuroleptics can aggravate or cause psychosis.

A few of the newer atypical neuroleptics have been found to cause metabolic changes in some individuals. The most common problems are development of diabetes mellitus and weight gain. Occasionally the elevation of the blood sugar can be sudden and severe, raising the need to check blood sugar, blood fats, and other chemistries.

Several of the neuroleptics block the appetite turn-off switch (the HT2 receptor) to varying degrees, which in turn can lead to gain in weight. Although weight gain ignored can lead to very severe obesity, weight gain appropriately addressed can be corrected. To bring about the necessary control of weight, the physician may have to prescribe diet, nutritional counseling, exercise program, and in rare instances even appetite suppressants.

Dopamine System Drugs (Blockers)

Drug Brand	Generic	Units in MG	Therapeutic Equivalence	Usual Daily Dose MGs	Rate of Dose Change MGs per	Age Approved*
Thorazine	(chlorpromazine)	10, 25, 30 100, 200	50	30–200	20–50/3 days	6 months
Mellaril	(thioridazine)	10, 15, 25 50, 100, 150	50	50–800	20–50/3 days	2 years
Trilafon	(perphenazine)	2, 4, 8, 16	5	4–16 (32 max)	2/3 days	12 years
Stelazine	(trifluoperazine)	1, 2, 5, 10	2.5	2.15 (40 max)	5/3 days	6 years
Navane	(thiothixene)	1, 2, 5, 10, 20	2.5	3–15 (60 max)	5/week	12 years
Haldol	(haloperidol)	.5, 1, 2, 5, 10, 20	1	1–6 (30 max)	.5/week	3 years
Prolixin	(fluphenazine)	1, 2.5, 5, 10	1	2.5–30 (40 max)	1/4 days	16 years
Orap	(pimozide)	1, 2	5	1–3 (10 max)	.5/3 days	12 years
Clozaril	(clozapine)	25, 30	75	50–450 (900 max)	100/week	16 years
Risperdal	(risperidone)	.25, .5, 1, 2, 3, 4	1	1.5–6	.5/week	15 years
Zyprexa	(olanzapine)	2.5, 5, 7.5, 10, 15	3.5	5–20	.5/week	17 years
Seroquel	(quetiapine)	25, 100, 200	50	75, 750	50/2 days	17 years
Geodon	(ziprasidone)	20, 40, 60, 80	50	40–160	40–80/weeks	18 years
Abilify	(aripiprazole)	10, 15, 20, 30	?	10–30	10/2 weeks	18 years
Loxitane	(loxapine)	5, 10, 25, 50	20	60–100	10/3 days	16 years

* The age of approved use is set by the Food and Drug Administration. This means studies sufficient to prove both safety and effectiveness have not been carried out in children and youth younger than this age.

Serotonin System

From an evolutionary aspect, serotonin is the oldest neurotransmitter. In mammals it originates in the raphe nucleus located in the core of the brain stem. During the development of the fetal brain, serotonin plays an important role in the migration of neurons to their proper position, thus allowing them to make correct connections. Serotonin neurons have a wide distribution throughout the whole brain. They connect to norepinephrine and dopamine neurons and can thereby modify their function. The serotonin system has the optimal strategic position for control, coordination, and

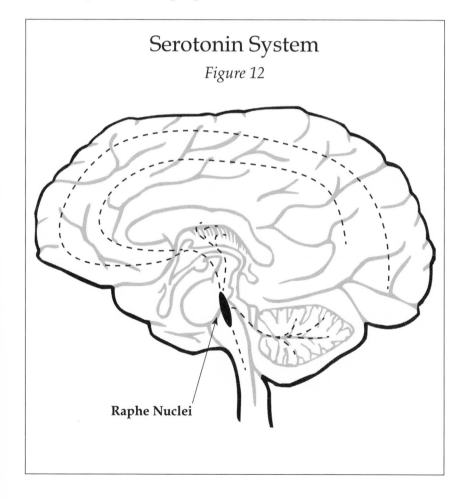

Serotonin System
Figure 12

Raphe Nuclei

integration of brain functions. It is no wonder that medications affecting the serotonin system have been helpful in a wide variety of disorders — i.e. anxiety, panic attack, depression, aggressions, obsessive compulsive, and eating disorders.

Serotonin is synthesized from the amino acid tryptophan. This process is relatively slow and inefficient when compared to the biosynthesis of the evolutionary new transmitters such as glutamate. As a result, serotonin stores can be depleted. With sleep, exhausted stores are regenerated to supply adequate levels for the activities of the next day.

Lower levels of serotonin are associated with:
- disrupted sleep, fragmented sleep, less REM sleep
- depression
- suicide
- violence
- increased appetite for carbohydrates
- increased risk of dying after a heart attack
- antisocial (psychopathic) personality disorder

"Higher" levels of serotonin are associated with:
- better impulse control
- reduced depression
- better mood
- better socialization
- avoidance of harm

There are many distinct receptors for serotonin, each of which is capable of producing a different effect when stimulated. So far 7 different groups have been identified and labeled with the abbreviation of the chemical name for serotonin 5 HT (5 hydroxytryptamine)

Serotonin receptors are distributed throughout the whole body but only those involved with brain function are listed:

5HT–1A

- inhibits neuronal activity and has a calming effect
- anti-depressant effect
- as an auto-receptor decreases serotonin release

5HT-2A

- stimulation by LSD ("acid") produces psychosis
- blocking of receptor by some neuroleptics reduces psychosis
- Stimulation important in regulating appetite
- Blockage results in uncontrolled appetite and weight gain

5HT6

- anti psychotic medications strongly bind to and block this receptor

Selective serotonin reuptake inhibitors (SSRIs) are a class of drugs which increases the amount of serotonin in the synapse by inhibiting its reuptake and removal.

These drugs have a number of advantages in that they are:

1.) Effective

2.) Accompanied by fewer side effects

3.) Administered once a day

4.) Relatively safe

5.) Much less lethal in deliberate overdosing

6.) Useful for a large number of disorders

Selective Serotonin Reuptake Inhibitors

Description

A class of drugs, SSRIs "selectively" increases serotonin

Prozac (fluoxetine)	Luvox (fluvoxamine)
Zoloft (sertraline)	Celexa (citalopram)
Paxil (paroxetine)	Lexapro (escitalopram)

Mechanism of Action

Inhibiting the transport system for the reuptake of serotonin increases the amount of serotonin in the synapse.

Indications and Uses

This group of medications has been found useful in a large number of disorders: depression, anxiety, panic attacks, obsessive compulsive disorder (OCD), eating disorders, anorexia nervosa, bulimia, stereotyptic movements, aggression, post traumatic stress disorder (PTSD). While non-approved uses are common, the Food and Drug Administration (FDA) has set the approved uses for the following drugs in adults.

Prozac	depression, OCD, bulimia, irritable bowel
Zoloft	depression, OCD, panic disorder, PTSD
Paxil	depression, OCD, panic disorder
Luvox	OCD
Celexa	depression

Prozac (fluoxetine) is the only SSRI approved for treating depression in children.

Side Effects

Common side effects include nausea, anorexia, weight gain, weight loss, diarrhea, insomnia, sleepiness, dry mouth. The side effect problems are generally milder and better tolerated. Sexual function can be affected in adolescents.

Warnings

These drugs cannot be used with, or soon after, monamine oxidase inhibitors.

Do not abruptly stop any SSRI antidepressant. Discontinuation must be under medical supervision so as not to increase risk of suicide.

What Else You Need to Know

Bipolar II illness commonly presents with depression and may be diagnosed as depression. When the depression is treated with SSRIs alone without the protection of a mood stabilizer, a serious manic episode could be induced. The same could be said for other antidepressants as well.

Drug interactions with Luvox cause significant increases in the blood levels of theophylline and benzodiazepine tranquilizers.

The Food and Drug Administration had issued warnings about possible increased suicidal thinking and suicidal attempts in clinical trials of eight SSRIs in children with depression. With recent allegations of undue pharmaceutical influence on the Agency it's response was to issue a severe "black box" (may cause death) warning for SSRIs.

A child who is treated may become energized before coming fully out of this depression and have a new capability to act on his suicidal thoughts. When SSRIs start working the family and friends may feel the child does not require the same intensive support. Some children may be very sensitive to the leveling off of support and become more depressed.

Children who demonstrate increased irritability or agitation in the first 6 to 8 weeks of starting treatment may be increased risk of suicide.

What is known is that:

1) SSRIs are potent medications that require close supervision,

2) SSRIs are very effective antidepressants,

3) Suicidal thinking and attempts are inherent in major depression,

4) Suicide is the 3rd leading cause of death in adolescents,

5) Further studies are needed to answer questions, about safety and accurately determining the benefit to risk ratio of using antidepressants in children.

"Selective" Serotonin Reuptake Inhibitors "SSRIs"

Drug	Unit MG	Usual Dose MG	Neuromodulations			Clinical Use Comments
			Sero.	Nor.	Dopa.	
Prozac (fluoxetine) liquid > 17	10, 20, 40	5–40 (60 max)	++++	+	0	depression, OCD, Tourette's bulimia, premenstral syndrome secondarily for ADHD Comment: 6 weeks for effect
Zoloft (sertraline) > 6	25, 50, 100	50–200	++++	+	+	OCD, depression, panic disorders, PTSD, selective mutism Comment: 1-2 weeks for effect
Paxil (paroxetine)	10, 20, 30, 40	20–40 (60 max)	++++	+	+	OCD, depression, panic disorder Comment: 1 week for effect
Luvox (fluvoxamine)	25, 50, 100	50–200 (300 max)	+++	0	0	OCD, secondarily for anxiety disorder Comment: 2 weeks for effect Caution: potentiates benzodiazepines
Celexa (citalopram)	10, 20, 40	10–20 (40 max)	++++	+	+	depression
Lexapro (escitalopram)	5, 10, 20	5–10 (20 max)	++++	+	+	depression, anxiety disorder. Must taper off to avoid anxiety and irritability.

SIDE EFFECTS: GI: nausea, vomiting, diarrhea, constipation CNS: anxiety, somnolence insomnia AUTONOMIC: sweating, dry mouth, abnrmal ejaculaion, dizziness

Atypical Serotonin Antidepressants
Desyrel (trazodone), Serzone (nefazodone)

Description

Desyrel is triazolopyride, a distinct chemical developed by Bristol-Myers-Squibb as an antidepressant. In an attempt to decrease side-effects alteration of the molecule formed nefazodone, now marketed as Serzone.

Mechanism of Action

Both medications have the same actions to increase serotonin by weakly blocking its reuptake, and blocking 5HT1 auto-receptors. Blocking of 5HT2 receptors enhances the antidepressant and anti-anxiety effects.

Indications and Uses

Both medications have been used for mild depression, anxiety, aggression, and bulimia. Desyrel with greater sedation is used for insomnia.

Side Effects

Each can produce mild stomach upset, nausea, headache, and sedation. Desyrel also has alpha1 blocking effects which can cause dry mouth, dizziness from a drop in blood pressure when standing, and painful swelling of the penis.

Monitoring

Blood pressure should be checked for Desyrel. Serzone requires periodic liver function testing.

Warnings

Serzone has caused (rare) liver damage severe enough to cause **DEATH.**

What Else You Need to Know

Canada has withdrawn Serzone from its market because the sever liver damage was unpredictable.

Desyrel is non-addicting and useful as a tranquilizer or sleeping medication in youth prone to addiction.

Atypical Serotonin Antidepressants

Drug	Units in MGs	Usual Daily Dose MGs	Ususal # Doses/Day	Rate of Dose Change	Approved for Use in Ages
Desyrel (trazodone)	50, 100, 150	start 50 50–200 400 max	2–3 times	50 mg/3days	<18 years
Serzone (nefazodone)	50, 100, 150 200, 250	start 50 150–300 600 max	2–3 times	50 mg/4days	<18 years

Mixed: Tricyclic Antidepressants

Description

Imipramine was the first successful antidepressant It was released in the early 1960s and soon followed by subsequent derivatives. Because of the chemical three ring structure, this class of medications has been called "tricyclics" and includes:

Tofranil	(imipramine)	Norpramin	(desipramine)
Pamelor	(nortriptyline)	Pertofrane	(desipramine)
Elavil	(amitriptyline)	Anafranil	(clomipramine)
		Sinequan	(doxepin)

Mechanism of Action

The tricyclics are non-selective serotonin inhibitors in that they also inhibit the reuptake of norepinephrine. Increased serotonin and norepinephrine both contribute to an antidepressant effect. Alpha 1 receptors are affected — their blocking is responsible for the undesired fall in blood pressure. Blocking of histamine receptors is responsible for the antihistamine side effects.

Indications and Uses

Primary use has been for treatment of depression. Other uses include anxiety disorder, panic attack. ADHD, obsessive compulsive disorder, bulimia, agoraphobia, adjunct for movement disorder, Tourette's syndrome, bed wetting.

Side Effects

Alpha 1 blocking can cause a drop in blood pressure with light headedness, dizziness, or fainting, rapid pulse and heart rhythm changes. Histamine and muscarinic choline receptors are blocked which can cause dry mouth, constipation, urinary retention, visual disturbances, tiredness, fatigue. Seizures can occur and mania can be precipitated.

Warnings

Electrical disturbances in the heart, indicated by prolongation of the QT interval on the electrocardiogram, can predispose to life threatening arrhythmia (of greatest concern with desipramine and nortriptyline). SEIZURES can occur.

What Else You Need to Know

The surge of estrogen in early adolescent girls can completely block the antidepressant effect.

Tricyclic Antidepressants

Drug	Advantages	Norepinephrine Effect	Dopamine Effect	Serotonin Effect
Anafranil (clomipramine)	decreased repetitive movements in autism decrease repetitive movements and thoughts in OCD	++	0	+++
Elavil, Endep (amitriptyline)	useful in pain control	+	0	++
Norpramin Pertofrane (desipramine)	decreases tics in Tourette's and effective in co-existing ADHD as well	+++	0	+
Trofanil (imipramine)	improves bed wetting, and night terrors	+	0	++
Pamelor (nortriptyline)	decreases tics in Tourette's and effective in co-existing ADHD as well	++	0	+
Sinequan (doxepin)	calming effect	+	0	++

Tricylic Antidepressants

Drug	Dose MG Unit	Usual Daily Dose MG	Approved Age	Clinical Use / Cautions
Tofranil (imipramine)	10, 25, 50	30–100	> 6 years	depression, enuresis, ADHD, bulimia, anxiety caution: cardiac arrhythmia
Pamelor (nortriptyline)	10, 25, 50	30–100	> 18 years	depression, ADHD with depression ADHD with Tourette's
Elavil, Endep (amitriptyline)	10, 25, 50, 75	30–100	> 12 years	depression, pain control
Norpramin Pertofrane (desipramine)	10, 25, 50, 75	25–150	> 18 years	depression, ADHD with depression ADHD with Tourette's, bulimia
Anafranil (clomipramine)	25, 50, 75	25–200	> 10 years	obsessive compulsive disorder, panic attack. Stereotypies in autism, agoraphobia. Caution: seizure
Sinequan (doxepin)	10, 25, 50, 75 100, 150	10–150		depression, anxiety, bed wetting, over stimulated GI tract, ulcer, irritable bowel

SIDE EFFECTS: CNS: drowsiness, incoordination, confusion, insomnia, nightmares, anxiety, seizures AUTONOMIC: dry mouth, blurred vision, constipation, change in libido CAUTION: EKG screening test before use Rare blood dyscrasia – monitor complete blood count (CBC) CNS = Central nervous system (the brain)

Mixed (Serotonin and Norepinephrine) Antidepressant: Cymbalta (duloxetine)

Description

Cymbalta is a new antidepressant in its own thiophenepropyl-amine class.

Mechanism of Action

Serotonin and norepinephrine are both increased by selective blocking of their reuptake systems.

Indications and Uses

Primarily used for major depression. Also has proved effective in the management of pain stemming from diabetic peripheral neuropathy.

Side Effects

Dizzyness, nausea, vomiting, constipation, irritability, nightmares, insomnia, somnolence, headache, inflammation of the liver, low blood sugar, pain with urination, and parasthesias can occur.

Monitoring

Periodic liver function and blood sugar tests are indicated. Blood pressure and pulse should be checked regularly.

Warning

As with the SSRIs, the FDA has put out suicide risk warnings (see p.67). Can not be used within 2-3 weeks of a monoamine oxidase inhibitor.

What Else You Need to Know

No studies have been done on persons younger than 18 years old.

Mixed (Serotonin and Norepinephrine) Antidepressant: Effexor (venlafaxine)

Description

Effexor is phenlethylamine, a structurally novel antidepressant.

Mechanism of Action

Primary effects are a strong inhibition of both serotonin and norepinephrine reuptake. It also has a weak inhibitory effect on dopamine reuptake.

Indications and Uses

Treatment of major depression is its primary use. It has also been proved of value in generalized anxiety disorder. Several studies indicate it has been very useful in ADHD.

Side Effects

Anxiety, nervousness, insomnia, and elevation of blood pressure may occur in those sensitive to the norepinephrine effect. Somnolence, dizziness, nausea, loss of appetite, and mania have not been infrequent.

Monitoring

Blood pressure should be measured.

Warnings

Caution in use with seizure disorder. As with SSRIs FDA has put out suicide risk warnings (discussion p.67)

Mixed (Serotonin and Norepinephrine) Antidepressant: Remeron (mirtazapine)

Description

Remeron is an antidepressant in its own separate piperazine chemical class.

Mechanism of Action

The drug's primary antidepressant effects are due to increased norepinephrine (caused by alpha 2 adrenergic blocking) and increased serotonin released when alpha 2 inhibitors are blocked. Blocking of histamine 1 receptors produces strong antihistamine effects of sedation and calming. Blocking of 5HT2 receptor predisposes to weight gain.

Indications and Uses

Primary use is for major, atypical and seasonal depression. Has also been effectively used in anxiety and panic disorders. Strong norepinephrine effects have been useful in ADHD. Antihistamine activity has benefitted bed-wetting and sleep disturbances.

Side Effects

Somnolence, sedation, dry mouth, constipation and weight gain. Some instances of dizziness particularly if there are blood pressure drops when standing up.

Monitoring

Blood pressure measurements to determine any unwanted elevation or lowering. When an infection is present a blood test to measure white blood cells may be indicated to detect the rare (one per thousand) occurrence of lowering the number of white blood cells.

Warning

Cannot be used within 2-3 weeks of taking a monoamine oxidate inhibitor. As with SSRIs FDA suicide risk warning (discussion p. 67).

What Else You Need to Know

Elevations of serum cholesterol and triglycerides can occur. While used extensively in adults no controlled studies in children have been reported.

Mixed (Serotonin & Norepinephrine) Antidepressants

Drug	Units in MGs	Usual Daily Dose MGs	Norepinephrine Effects	Serotonin Effects
Cymbalta (duloxetine)	20, 30, 60	40–60	++	++
Effexor (venlafaxine)	25, 37.5, 50, 100	75–225	+++	++++
Remeron (mirtazapine)	15, 30, 45	15–45	++	++

Mixed (Serotonin, Norepinephrine, Dopamine) Antidepressant: Wellbutrin (bupropion)

Description

Wellbutrin is an antidepressant in its own separate aminoketone class and is not chemically related to other antidepressants

Mechanism of Action

The drug has a mild inhibition of the reuptake on all three neuromodulators, — norepinephrine, dopamine and serotonin.

Indications and Uses

Wellbutrin is indicated for the treatment of depression. It has been found to be effective in the treatment of attention deficit hyperactivity disorder either alone or when accompanied by conduct disorder.

Side Effects

Agitation, insomnia, and weight gain are common. Wellbutrin can cause seizures. Low incidence of sexual side effects.

Rare side effects include psychosis, confusion mania, hallucinations and paranoia. These phenomena generally clear with discontinuing, or reducing the dose.

Monitoring

No special testing required.

Warnings

Should not be used in anyone with a seizure disorder.

What Else You Need to Know

Do not use with Zyban, which is another form of bupropion, marketed to stop smoking.

Wellbutrin (bupropion)

Advantages	Disadvantages	Norepinephrine Effect	Dopamine Effect	Serotonin Effect
useful for ADHD + depression + conduct disorder + substance abuse	increase tics increase seizures	++	++	+

Units in MG	Usual Daily Dose	Duration Effect	Usual Doses/Day	Rate of Dose Change
75, 100, 100, 150, SR	200–400	8–12 hours	2 times	50–100 / 4 weeks

SIDE EFFECTS: headache 26%, dry mouth 17%, nausea 13%, insomnia 11%, anxiety 5%, agitation 3%. Serious side effects but rare: seizures 0.4%. To minimize risk of seizures use SR (sustained release) formulation. Approved for age 18.

Mixed (Serotonin, Norepinephrine, Dopamine) Antidepressants: Monoamine Oxidase Inhibitors

Description

Type A monomine oxidise inhibitors increase the amines dopamine, serotonin, and norepinephrine non-selectively. Drugs in this class include:

Nardil   (phenelzine)

Parnate   (tranylcypromine)

Marplan (isocarboxazid)

Mechanism of Action

By inhibiting the enzymatic breakdown and destruction of amines the activity of pharmocologically active amines dopamine, serotonin, and norepinephrine are increased.

Indications and Uses

These medications have been used primarily in the treatment of depression which has been resistant to all other types of antidepressants. Because of severe risks, if taken with a host of other medications, or if taken with a prohibited food, their use is severely restricted. They have limited but effective use in bulimia and some forms of ADHD.

Side Effects

Common side effects include: drop in blood pressure with standing up, headache, drowsiness, disturbed sleep, fatigue, constipation, dry mouth, weight gain, anxiety, euphoria, and visual disturbances.

Warnings

Severe elevations of blood pressure, hypertensive crisis, can result if taken with incompatible drugs or restricted foods. Use of these medications is limited to responsible, reliable individuals. Their use is usually restricted to adults. Only Nardil has received FDA approval for ages as young as 16.

Drugs prohibited while taking MAOI's include sympathomimetic drugs, often found in decongestant, asthma and "cold and allergy" medications, anaesthesia, narcotic pain medications, blood pressure medications, diuretics ("water pills"), stimulants (methylphenidate, amphetamines) and any other antidepressant.

Food that must be avoided are aged cheeses, yogurt, sour cream, pickled herring, anchovies, Genoa salami, hard salami, pepperoni, lebanon bologna, caviar liver, figs, dried fruits, bananas, raspberries, avocado, fava beans, sauerkraut, soy sauce, beer, wine, liqueurs, too much caffeine, and **chocolate.**

What Else You Need to Know

These medications are not a first or second line choice, but are restricted to reliable individuals who have not responded to any other agents. Special consultation, for a thorough and careful analysis, is required for the consideration of their use.

```
┌─────────────────────────────────┐
│          Inhibitors             │
│                                 │
│        Benzodiazepines          │
│                                 │
│         Antihistamine           │
│                                 │
│           Atypical              │
└─────────────────────────────────┘
```

Benzodiazepines

Description

Benzodiazepine is a large family of medications that have a calming, anxiety-reducing effect. They share very similar side-effects, but have a wide range in their duration of action which determines their practical use. Drugs of shorter duration are often referred to as tranquilizers, while those of longer duration may be called hypnotics or sleeping medications. Members of the benzodiazepine family are:

Halcion	(triazolam)	Valium	(diazepam)
Xanax	(alprazolam)	Restoril	(temazepam)
Ativan	(lorazepam)	Tranxene	(clorazepate)
Librium	(chlordiazepoxide)	Klonopin	(clonazepam)

Mechanism of Action

Brain cells (neurons) function by generating and conducting electrical energy. Like other electrical circuits they are equipped with separate switches (chemical receptors) to turn on (stimulators) and to turn off (inhibitors). GABA is the nervous system's natural chemical inhibitor that decreases nerve cell (neuron) activity.

The pharmocological activity of all benzodiazepine medications takes place at the GABA receptor (turn off switch) by enhancing the effect of GABA. Different types of GABA receptors have been discovered and are thought to affect different functions — such as: decrease in anxiety, reduce wakefulness, inhibit seizures, stop muscle spasm. One benzodiazepine may have greater effectiveness at one type of GABA receptor than another, and thus have different effects and uses.

Indications and Uses

Antianxiety medications are useful in reducing excessive worrying, nervousness and fears. They are helpful in many disorders.

1) Anxiety Disorders: school phobia, separation anxiety, panic attacks, night terrors, environmental stresses.

2) Behavioral Disorders: impulsivity, aggression, self injurious behavior, conduct disorders, sleepwalking, adolescent adjustment disorder.

3) Medical Uses: seizure disorder, muscle relaxant

Side Effects

Side effects are generally related to decreased or slowed brain activity: over-sedation, fatigue, drowsiness, slurred speech, loss of balance, blurred vision, loss of memory, depression, confusion and coma.

Monitoring

No special laboratory tests are required.

Warnings

ADDICTING! DO NOT STOP SUDDENLY!

Overdoses are serious — coma and DEATH possible

There is a tendency for tolerance whereby the child becomes "used to" the medication and larger doses are required to achieve the same beneficial effect. The medications are addicting, and can be abused. The medications need to be stopped gradually by tapering off. Suddenly stopping could produce withdrawal and severe SEIZURES.

Halcion has caused temporary loss of memory (antegrade amnesia) with resultant acute disorientation.

What Else You Need to Know

Paradoxical effect:

> Inhibition of a brain cell which stimulates an activity, will reduce that activity. But some brain cells function to control and inhibit other neurons. When these inhibitory neurons are turned off, those neurons previously controlled become more active and may become too excited. This excitement and overactivity is an opposite or paradoxical effect.

> Marked disinhibiton, loss of control, acute excitement, aggression, rage, and nightmares are paridoxical effects. If this happens STOP the medicine and CALL your child's doctor.

Always double check to insure that your child's health professionals (pharmacist, nurse, physician) have not mis-heard or misinterpreted either Klonopin or clonidine, and confused them.

"Minor" Tranquilizers – Benzodiazepines

Drug	How Supplied MG	Usual Daily Dose MG	Duration of Action (Hours)	Usual Doses/Day	Approved for Use in Ages
Halcion (triazolam)	.125, .25	.125–.25	Ultra Short 1.5–4	1 bedtime	> 18 years
Xanax (alprazolam)	.5, 1	.5–4	Short 3	3–4 times	> 18 years
Ativan (lorazepam)	.5, 1, 2	1–4	Medium 4–8	3–4 times	> 12 years
Librium (chlordiazepoxide)	5, 10, 20	15–40	Medium 4–6	3–4 times	> 6 years
Valium (diazepam)	2, 5, 10	2–15	Medium–Long	2 times	> 6 months
Restoril (temazepam)	7.5, 15, 30	15–30	Medium	1 bedtime	> 18 years
Tranxene (clorazepate)	3.75, 7.5, 15, SD 11.25, 22.5	13–60	Medium–Long	2 times	> 9 years
Klonopin (clonazepam)	.5, 1	.25–2	Medium–Long	2 times	> 7 years

Antihistamines
Atarax, Vistaril (hydroxyzine), Benadryl (diphenhydramine) Periactin (cyproheptadine)

Description

Antihistamines are a class of medications that were designed to treat allergies. One of the unwanted side-effects, sedation, has proved quite useful in providing safe tranquilization in children.

Mechanism of Action

These antihistamines bind to the H1 histamine receptor.

Indications

Antihistamines generally are safe and are often used either as a mild tranquilizer to reduce anxiety or nervousness, but may also be effective in inducing sleep.

Side Effects

Sleepiness, decreased attention, dry mouth, blurred vision, dizziness, constipation, uncoordinated movements.

Monitoring

No special laboratory monitoring required.

Warnings

- Can worsen asthma.

- Very rarely can have paradoxical excitement with uncontrollable behavior, and even convulsions.

- Can worsen glaucoma (increased fluid pressure in the eye).

Antihistamines

Drug	How Supplied MG	Usual Daily Dose Doses/Day	Usual # MG in 24 hours
Atarax, Vistaril (hydroxyzine)	10, 25, 50, 1000	10–100	3–4
Benadryl (diphenhydramine)	12.5, 25	12.5–100	1–3
Periactin (cyproheptadine)	4	2–16	2–3
Phenergan (promethazine)	12.5, 25, 50	12.5–50	2–3

Atypical "Minor" Tranquilizer
BuSpar (buspirone)

Description

BuSpar is an antianxiety medication. It differs from the benzodiazepines in that it is milder, much safer, but shares many of the same uses.

Mechanism of Action

BuSpar binds to and moderately stimulates the 5 HTIA receptor to cause relaxation and calming.

Indications and Uses

Not as strong or as effective as the benzodiazepines in the treatment of more severe anxiety and behavioral disorders. It is useful in mild generalized anxiety, school phobia, anxiety mixed with depression of substance abuse. Has also been used in treatment of aggression and self-injurious behavior. It is not useful for sleep disorders and has no anti-seizure activity.

Side Effects

BuSpar may cause restlessness, nervousness, headache, dizziness, nausea or trouble sleeping.

Monitoring

No specific testing required.

Warnings

Paradoxical effect can happen rarely with disinhibition, aggression, and uncontrollable behavior.

WHAT ELSE YOU NEED TO KNOW

- May work slowly and not reach effectiveness for 6 weeks.

- Be careful that buspirone is not confused with bupropion.

"Minor" Tranquilizer

Drug	How Supplied MG	Usual Daily Dose	Duration of Effect	Usual # Doses/Day	Approved for Use in Ages
BuSpar (buspirone)	5, 10, 15, 30	10–30 60 Max	3 hours initially, days eventually	2–3 times	> 18 years

+-------------------------------------+
| **Stabilizers** |
| |
| Anticonvulsants |
| |
| Lithium |
+-------------------------------------+

Anticonvulsants (Mood Stabilizers)

DESCRIPTION

The first medications used to prevent neurons from reacting to surrounding activity and electrical stimulation were used to control seizures and thus called anticonvulsants. The anticonvulsants most commonly used to stabilize mood are listed:

Carbatrol	(carbamazepine)	Lamictal	(lamotrigine)
Tegretol	(carbamazepine)	Neurontin	(gabapentin)
Depakene	(valproic acid)	Topamax	(topiramate)
Depakote	(divalproex)	Trileptal	(oxcarbazepine)

Mechanism of Action

The exact mechanism by which anticonvulsants electrically stabilize the neuron's cellular membrance and prevent the neurons from becoming activated is complex. Enhancement of inhibitors, direct anti-stimulant effects are combined with other mechanisms not fully understood.

Indications and Uses

These medications are used in bipolar disorder to decrease mood swings and prevent mania and depression. These medications are also effective in explosive behavioral disorders, severe aggression, conduct disorder and self-injurious behavior.

Neuralgia and other types of pain can be controlled with these medications.

New anti-depression effects have been discovered for Lamictal! With the recent FDA "black box" (may cause death) warnings for SSRIs and their known potential risk of precipitating mania, Lamictal is emerging as a drug of choice in bipolar illness with depression.

Side Effects — General

This group of medications share common side effects of tiredness and sleepiness as well as some behavioral problems of irritability and aggression. However, several side effects are seen only with a specific medication and require separate listings.

Side Effects

Carbatrol, Tegretol (carbamazepine)

Common: nausea, dizziness, sleepiness, double vision, clumsiness, hair loss

Behavioral: anxiety, agitation, irritability, impulsivity, aggression

Rare: severe skin rash, damage to bone marrow

Depakene (valproic acid) Depakote (divalproex)

Common: nausea, increased appetite, headache, weight gain, tiredness, menstrual changes, tremor, dizziness

Behavioral: irritability, increased aggression, somnolence

Rare: severe liver damage in children under 6, inflammation of pancreas, cystic enlargement of ovaries

Lamictal (lamotrigine)

Common: sleepiness, headache, unsteadiness, vision problems, nausea

Behavioral: anxiety, agitation

Rare: severe skin rash, liver inflamation

Neurontin (gabapentin) Gabitril (tiagabine)

Common: sleepiness, unsteadiness, fatigue, involuntary jerking movements of the eyes

Behavioral: temper tantrums, irritability, aggression

Rare: depression, abnormal thinking

Topamax (topiramate)

Common: sleepiness, confusion, nervousness, memory problems, shakiness, dizziness, sloved movements, unsteadiness, speech problems, disturbed vision

Behavioral: nervousness, anxiety, irritability

Rare: confusion

Periodic blood test for blood count and liver function testing is advisable.

Trileptal (oxcarbazepine)

Common: nausea, vomiting, fatigue, headach, dizziness, somnolence, double vision.

Behavioral: nervousness, emotional liability, anxiety, amnesia, insomnia

Rare: convulsions aggravated, low serum sodium

Monitoring

Periodic blood testing of liver function and complete blood count are required. Serum sodium needs to be monitored for Trileptal.

WARNINGS

Depakene (valproic acid) Depakote (divalproex)

Although rare, severe liver damage even resulting in DEATH has occurred. Children under the age of 2 are most susceptible but children under the age of 6 who are taking more than one medication are at risk.

Lamictal (lamotrigine)

Very severe allergic skin damage (Stevens—Johnson syndrome) occures in 0.8%. The reaction usually occurs within the first 2 months.

Tegretol, Carbatrol (carbamazepine)

Severe damage to bone marrow with resultant loss of red and white blood cells. This reaction can cause death. Very, very rare. Occurs one in 100,000 patients.

Trileptal (oxcarbazepine)

Low serum sodium (hyponatremia) may occur in 2–3%. This reaction can produce nausea, malaise, lethargy, confusion and increased or new seizures.

What Else You Need to Know

With individual sensitivity, or with too high a blood level, these medications can cause temporary problems with cerebellar function. This can result in dizziness, unstable walking, jerking movements of the eyes, problems with vision, gross impairment of coordination.

Lithium (Mood Stabilizier)

Description

Lithium is a naturally occurring salt that is marketed in different forms:

Eskalith   Lithobid   Lithium citrate syrup (liquid form)

Mechanism of Action

Lithium interferes with chemical cascade that effects gene turn on and gene turn off initiated by Dopamine. Another newly discovered effect of lithium is that it stimulates the production of a substance that restores well-being to neurons.

MEDICATIONS AND USES

Primary use has been in bipolar disorder to stabilize mood swings and has been a therapeutic mainstay of preventing recurrences with maintenance treatment. It has an anti-depression effect and lowers the risk of suicide. Other uses include aggression and tantrums.

SIDE EFFECTS

Weight gain, tiredness, weakness, headache, diarrhea, increased thirst, increased urination, nausea, dizziness, tremor, acne. Hair loss is rare.

MONITORING

Regular periodic blood tests are necessary to monitor the blood level of lithium. Kidney function tests are required regularly, but less often. Thyroid function may have to be checked.

WARNINGS

Build up of lithium in the blood can cause severe poisoning with nausea, vomiting, diarrhea, tremor, somnolence, coma and even DEATH. Kidney damage can result.

WHAT ELSE YOU NEED TO KNOW

Children under the age of 7 are much more prone to troublesome side-effects. Extreme variation in dietary intake of salt can cause blood levels of lithium to vary markedly. Excessive sweating with severe exercise, inadequate water intake, or exaggerated fluid loss, due to intestinal flu, can cause lithium toxicity. Consult your physician to know when lithium should be withheld.

Signs of too much lithium (toxicity) include fainting, staggering, irregular pulse, blurred vision, ringing in the ears, muscle twitching, fever, convulsions and loss of consciousness.

Mood Stabilizers and Anticonvulsants

Drug	How Supplied MG	Usual Daily Dose MG	Usual # Doses/Day	Approved for Use in Ages	Side Effects/ Monitoring
(lithium carb.) Eskalith Lithobid (lithium citrate)	300 300 300, 450 8/top liquid	600–1800	3–4 times 2 times	> 12 years	Diarrhea, vomiting, ataxia coarse tremor, drowsiness, impaired coordination. Monitor: serum level, kidney, thyroid
(valproic acid) Depakene	250	Min 7mg/lb Max 27mg/lb	2–4 times	> 16 years	Nausea, vomiting Sedation, depression,
(divalproex) Depakote	125,250 500				aggression, psychosis. Monitor: liver function
(carbamazepine) Tegretol Carbatrol	100,200 XR, 100, 200 XR, 400	2–25mg/lb 800–1200	4 times 2 times 2 times	> 6 years	Dizziness, drowsiness, ataxia, nausea, vomiting. Rare: aggression, mania. Monitor liver function-blood count
(gabapentin) Neurontin	100, 300 400, 600, 800	900–1800	3 times	> 12 years	Somnolence, fatigue, ataxia, nausea

(continues on next page)

Mood Stabilizers and Anticonvulsants *(continued)*

Drug	How Supplied MG	Usual Daily Dose MG	Usual # Doses/Day	Approved for Use in Ages	Side Effects/ Monitoring
(lamotrigine) Lamictal	5, 25, 100 150, 200	50–400 max 800	2 times		Somnolence, dizziness, ataxia antidepressant effect, nausea, Stevens-Johnson rash .1%
(topiramate) Topomax	25, 100 200	100–200 max 400	2 times		Impaired concentration, dizziness weight loss ataxia, speech problems, nausea. Monitor: liver function, blood count
(tiagabine) Gabitril	2, 4, 12 16, 20	4–28	2 times		Somnolence, dizziness, nausea, impaired concentration
(oxcarbazepine) Trileptal	150, 300, 600 300/tsp	900–1800	2times		Nausea, somnolence fatigue, ataxia, double vision. Monitor: serum sodium

Appendix

Internet Resources

American Academy of Child and
Adolescent Psychiatry
3615 Wisconsin Avenue, NW
Washington, DC 20016-3007
1-202-966-7300
www.aacap.org

The American Psychiatric
Association
1000 Wilson Blvd., Suite 1825
Arlington, VA 22209-3901
1-703-904-7300
www. parentsmedguide.org

Anxiety Disorders Association of
America (ADAA))
1900 Parklawn Drive
Rockville, MD 20852
1-301-231-9350
www.adaa.org

Autism Society of America
7910 Woodmont Avenue, Suite 300
Bethesda, MD 20814-3067
1-800-3-AUTISM
www.autism-society.org

Children and Adults With
Attention-Deficit Hyperactivity
Disorder (CHADD)
Hyperactivity Disorder (CHADD
8181 Professional Place, Suite 201
Landover, MD 20785
1-800-233-4050 (National Call Center)

Child & Adolescent Bipolar Foundation
1187 Wilmett Avenue
P.M.B. #331
Wilmette, IL 60091
1-847-256-8525
www.bpkids.org

Council of Educators for Students
With Disabilities
(OASIS)
9801 Anderson Mill Road, Suite 230
Austin, TX 78750
1-512-219-5043
www504idea.org

Federation of Families for
Children's Mental Health
1101 King Street, Suite 420
Alexandria, VA 22314
1-703-684-7710
www.ffcmh.org

NAMI New Jersey
1562 Route 130
North Brunswick, N.J. 08902
1-732-940-0991
www.naminj.org

National Alliance for the Mentally Ill
(NAMI)
Colonial Place Three
2107 Wilson Boulevard, Suite 300
Arlington, VA 22201
1-800-950-NAMI or 1-703-524-7600
www.nami.org

National Depressive and
Manic-Depressive Association
730 North Franklin Street, Suite 501
Chicago, IL 60610
1-312-642-0049
www.ndmda.org

National Institute of Mental Health
NIMH Public Inquires
6001 Executive Boulevard
Room 8184, MSC 9663
Bethesda, MD 20892
1-301-433-4513
www.nimh.gov

New Jersey Psychiatric Association
P.O. Box 8008
Bridgewater, N.J. 08807-8008
1-908-685-0650
www.psychnj.org

Online Asperger Syndrome
Information and Support
(OASIS)
www.aspergersyndrome.org

Tourette Syndrome Association
42-40 Bell Boulevard
Bayside, N.Y. 11361
1-718-224-2999
www.tsa-usa.org

Surgeon General's Report on Children's Mental Health

Overarching Vision

Mental health is a critical component of children's learning and general health. Fostering social and emotional health in children as a part of a healthy child development must therefore be a national priority. Both the promotion of mental health in children and the treatment of mental disorders should be major public health goals. To achieve these goals, the Surgeon General's National Action Agenda for Children's Mental Health takes as its guiding principles a commitment to:

1. Promoting the recognition of mental health as an essential part of child health;

2. Integrating family, child and youth-centered mental health services into all systems that serve children and youth;

3. Engaging families and incorporating the perspectives of children and youth in the development of all mental healthcare planning; and

4. Developing and enhancing a public-private health infrastructure to support these efforts to the fullest extent possible.

The Report Proposes a National Children's Mental Health Agenda with Eight Goals

Goals

1. Promote public awareness of children's mental health issues and reduce stigma associated with mental illness.

2 Continue to develop, disseminate, and implement scientifically proven prevention and treatment services in the field of children's mental health.

3. Improve the assessment of and recognition of mental health needs in children.

4. Eliminate racial/ethnic and socioeconomic disparities in access to mental healthcare services.

5. Improve the infrastructure for children's mental health services, including support for scientifically proven interventions across professions.

6. Increase access to and coordination and quality mental healthcare services.

7. Train frontline providers to recognize and manage mental health issues, and educate mental healthcare providers about scientifically proven prevention and treatment services.

8. Monitor the access to and coordination of quality mental healthcare services.

Bibliography

A.R. Damaso. "Descartes Error". New York: Putnam's Sons, 1994

M.K. Dulcan, D.R. Martini, M. Lake, "Concise Guide to Child and Adolescent Psychiatry" Third Edition. Washington, D.C.: American Psychiatric Publishing, 2003.

W.H. Green. "Child & Adolescent Clinical Psychopharmacology" Third Edition. Philadelphia: Lippincott Williams & Wilkins, 2001.

J.C. Harris. "Developmental Neuropsychiatry" Volume I. New York: Oxford University Press, 1995.

A.F. Schatzberg, J.O. Cole, C. DeBattista. "Manual of Clinical Psychopharmacology" Fourth Edition. Washington, D.C.: American Psychiatric Publishing, 2003.

D.J. Siegel. "The Developing Mind". New York: Guilford Press, 1999.

D.J. Siegel, M. Hartzell. "Parenting from the Inside Out" New York: Tarcher/Putnam, 2003.

M. Spitzer. "The Mind Within the Net". Cambridge, Ma.: The MIT Press, 1999.

T.E. Wilens. "Straight Talk about Psychiatric Medications for Kids". New York: Guilford Press, 2001.

Index of Medications

Brand names are capitalized, generic names are lower case.

fluvoxamine	65-68	Nefazodone	69-70
Focalin	50-51,53-54	Neurontin	91-94, 97
gabapentin	91-94, 97	Norpramin	71-74
Geodon	59-62	nortriptyline	71-74
guanfacine	39-40, 42-43	olanzapine	59-62
Halcion	83-86	Orap	59-62
Haldol	59-62	oxcarbazepine	59-62
haloperidol	59-62	Pamelor	71-74
hydroxyzine	87-88	Parnate	81-82
imipramine	71-74	paroxetine	65-68
Inderal	44-46	Paxil	65-68
isocarboxazid	81-82	pemoline	51-54
Klonopin	83-86	Periactin	87-88
Lamictal	91-94, 98	perphenazine	59-62
lamotrigine	91-94, 98	Pertofrane	71-74
Librium	83-86	phenelzine	81-82
Lexapro	65-68	Phenergan	87-88
lithium	95-97	pimozide	59-62
Lithobid	95-97	pindolol	44-46
lorazepam	83-86	Prolixin	59-62
loxapine	59-62	promethazine	87-88
Loxitane	59-62	propranolol	44-46
Luvox	65-68	Prozac	65-68
Marplan	81-82	quetiapine	59-62
Mellaril	59-62	reboxetine	42
Metadate	50-51, 53-54	Remeron	77-78
methylphenidate	50-51, 53-54	Restoril	83-86
mirtazapine	77-78	risperidone	59-62
nadolol	44-46	Risperdal	59-62
Nardil	81-82	Ritalin	50-51, 53-54
Navane	59-62	Seroquel	59-62

sertraline	65-68	Tranxene	83-86
Serzone	69-70	trazodone	69-70
Sinequan	71-74	triazolam	83-86
Stelazine	59-62	trifluoperazine	59-62
Strattera	41-43	Trilafon	59-62
Tegretol	91-94, 97	Trileptal	91-94, 98
temazepam	83-86	Valium	83-86
Tenex	39-40, 42-43	valproic acid	91-94, 98
Tenormin	44-46	venlafaxine	76, 78
thioridazine	59-62	Visken	44-46
thiothixine	59-62	Vistaril	87-88
Thorazine	59-62	Wellbutrin	79-80
tiagabine	91-94, 98	Xanax	83-86
Tofranil	71-74	ziprasidone	59-62
Topamax	91-94, 98	Zoloft	65-68
topiramate	91-94, 98	Zyban	79-80
tranylcypromine	81-82	Zyprexa	59-62

NAMI State Offices

Alabama
NAMI Alabama
6900 6th Avenue, South, Suite B
Birmingham, AL 35212-1902
Phone 1: (205) 833-8336
Phone 2: (800) 626-4199
Fax: (205) 833-8309
Email: office@namialabama.org

Alaska
NAMI Alaska
144 W 15th Ave
Anchorage, AK 99501-5106
Phone 1: (907) 277-1300
Phone 2: (800)478-4462
Fax: (907) 277-1400
Email: info@nami-alaska.org

Arizona
NAMI Arizona
2210 N 7th St
Phoenix, AZ 85006-1604
Phone 1: (602) 244-8166
Phone 2: (800) 626-5022
Fax: (602) 244-9264
Email: azami@azami.org

Arkansas
NAMI Arkansas
712 W 3rd Street, Suite 200
Little Rock, AR 72201-2222
Phone 1: (501) 661-1548
Phone 2: (800) 844-0381
Fax: (501) 664-0264

California
NAMI California
1010 Hurley Way, Ste 195
Sacramento, CA 95825-3218
Phone 1: (916) 567-0163
Fax: (916) 567-1757
Email: support@namicalifornia.org

Colorado
NAMI Colorado
1100 Fillmore Street, Ste. 201
Denver, CO 80206-3334
Phone 1: (303) 321-3104
Phone 2: (888) 566-6264
Fax: (303) 321-0912
Email: nami-co@nami.org

Connecticut
NAMI of Connecticut, Inc
30 Jordan Lane, 3rd Floor
Wethersfield, CT 06109
Phone 1: (860) 882-0236
Phone 2: (800) 215-3021
Fax: (860) 882-0240
Email: namict@namict.org

Delaware
NAMI Delaware
2400 W 4th St Plaza, Ste. 5
Wilmington, DE 19805-3306
Phone 1: (302) 427-0787
Phone 2: (888) 427-2643
Fax: (302) 427-2075
Email: namide@namide.org

District of Columbia
NAMI DC
422 8th St SE, 2nd Floor
Washington, DC 20003-2832
Phone 1: (202) 546-0646
Fax: (202) 546-6817
Email: namidc@aol.com

Florida
NAMI Florida
911 E Park Ave
Tallahassee, FL 32301-2646
Phone 1: (850) 671-4445
Phone 2: (877) 626-4352
Fax: (850) 671-5272
Email: lynne@namifl.org

Georgia
NAMI Georgia
3050 Presidential Dr, Suite 202
Atlanta, GA 30340-3916
Phone 1: (770) 234-0855
Phone 2: (800) 728-1052
Fax: (770) 234-0237
Email: nami-ga@nami.org

Hawaii
NAMI Hawaii State
84-1170 Farrington Hwy, C-1
Waianae, HI 96792-2025
Phone 1:(808) 695-9379
Fax: (808) 585-7843
Email: namihawaii@hawaii.rr.com

Idaho
NAMI Idaho
PO Box 68
362 West St
Albion, ID 83311-0068
Phone 1: (208) 673-6672
Phone 2: (800) 572-9940
Fax: (208) 673-6685
Email: namiid@atcnet.net

Illinois
NAMI Illinois
218 W Lawrence Ave
Springfield, IL 62704-2612
Phone 1: (217) 522-1403
Phone 2: (800) 346-4572
Fax: (217) 522-3598
Email: namiil@sbcglobal.net

Indiana
NAMI Indiana
PO Box 22697
Indianapolis, IN 46222-0697
Phone 1: (317) 925-9399
Phone 2: (800) 677-6442
Fax: (317) 925-9398
Email: nami-in@nami.org

Iowa
NAMI Iowa
Attn.: Margaret Stout
5911 Meredith Drive, Ste. E
Des Moines, IA 50322-1903
Phone 1: (515) 254-0417
Phone 2: (800) 417-0417
Fax: (515) 254-1103
Email: amiiowa@aol.com

Kansas

NAMI Kansas
112 SW 6th Ave, Suite 505
PO Box 675
Topeka, KS 66601-0675
Phone 1: (785) 233-0755
Phone 2: (800) 539-2660
Fax: (785) 233-4804
Email: namikansas@nami.org

Kentucky

NAMI Kentucky
10510 Lagrange Rd
Bldg 103
Louisville, KY 40223-1277
Phone 1: (502) 245-5284
Phone 2: (800) 257-5081
Fax: (502) 245-6390
Email: namiky@nami.org

Louisiana

NAMI Louisiana
11762 S Harrells Ferry Rd, Ste D
Baton Rouge, LA 70816-2398
Phone 1: (225) 292-6928
Phone 2: (888) 343-5864
Fax: (225) 368-0055
Email: namilouisiana@bellsouth.net

Maine

NAMI Maine
1 Bangor St
Augusta, ME 04330-4701
Phone 1: (207) 622-5767
Phone 2: (800) 464-5767
Fax: (207) 621-8430
Email: namime@gwi.net

Maryland

NAMI Maryland
804 Landmark Dr
Suite 122
Glen Burnie, MD 21061-4486
Phone 1: (410) 863-0470
Phone 2: (800) 467-0075
Fax: (410) 863-0474
Email: amimd@aol.com

Massachusetts

NAMI Massachusetts
400 West Cummings Park, Ste 6650
Woburn, MA 01801-6528
Phone 1: (781) 938-4048
Phone 2: (800) 370-9085
Fax: (781) 938-4069
Email: namimass@aol.com

Michigan

NAMI Michigan
921 N Washington Ave
Lansing, MI 48906-5137
Phone 1: (517) 485-4049
Phone 2: (800) 331-4264
Fax: (517) 485-2333
Email: namimichigan@acd.net

Minnesota

NAMI Minnesota
800 Transfer Rd
Suite 7A
Saint Paul, MN 55114-1422
Phone 1: (651) 645-2948
Phone 2: (888) 473-0237
Fax: (651) 645-7379
Email: nami-mn@nami.org

Mississippi
NAMI Mississippi
411 Briarwood Dr, Ste 401
Jackson, MS 39206-3058
Phone 1: (601) 899-9058
Phone 2: (800) 357-0388
Fax: (601) 956-6380
Email: namimiss1@aol.com

Missouri
NAMI Missouri
1001 Southwest Blvd, Ste E
Jefferson City, MO 65109-2501
Phone 1: (573) 634-7727
Phone 2: (800) 374-2138
Fax: (573) 761-5636
Email: mocami@aol.com

Montana
NAMI Montana
Mihelish's Residence
554 Toole Ct
Helena, MT 59602-6946
Phone 1: (406) 443-7871
Phone 2: (888) 280-6264
Fax: (406) 862-6357
Email: namimt@ixi.net

Nebraska
NAMI Nebraska
1941 S 42nd St, Ste 517–Center Mall
Omaha, NE 68105-2986
Phone 1: (877) 463-6264
Phone 2: (402) 345-8101
Fax: (402) 346-4070
Email: nami.nebraska@nami.org

Nevada
NAMI Nevada
1170 Curti Dr
Reno, NV 89502-1738
Phone 1: (775) 329-3260
Fax: (775) 329-1618
Email: joetyler@sdi.net

New Hampshire
NAMI New Hampshire
15 Green St
Concord, NH 03301-4020
Phone 1: (603) 225-5359
Phone 2: (800) 242-6264
Fax: (603) 228-8848
Email: naminh@naminh.org

New Jersey
NAMI New Jersey
1562 US Highway 130
North Brunswick, NJ 08902-3004
Phone 1: (732) 940-0991
Fax: (732) 940-0355
Email: naminj@optonline.net

New Mexico
NAMI New Mexico
PO Box 3086
6001 Marble NE Ste. 8
Albuquerque, NM 87190-3086
Phone 1: (505) 260-0154
Fax: (505) 260-0342
Email: ejonesnami@aol.com

New York
NAMI – NYS
260 Washington Ave
Albany, NY 12210-1312
Phone 1: (518) 462-2000
Phone 2: (800) 950-3228
Fax: (518) 462-3811
Email: naminys@naminys.org

North Carolina
NAMI North Carolina
309 W Millbrook Rd, Ste 121
Raleigh, NC 27609-4394
Phone 1: (919) 788-0801
Phone 2: (800) 451-9682
Fax: (919) 788-0906
Email: mail@naminc.org

North Dakota
NAMI North Dakota
PO Box 6016
Minot, ND 58702-6016
Phone 1: (701) 852-8202
Fax: (701) 725-4334
Email: jsabol@srt.com

Ohio
NAMI Ohio
747 East Broad Street
Columbus, OH 43205
Phone 1: (614) 224-2700
Phone 2: (800) 686-2646
Fax: (614) 224-5400
Email: amiohio@amiohio.org

Oklahoma
NAMI Oklahoma
500 N Broadway Ave, Ste 100
Oklahoma City, OK 73102-6200
Phone 1: (405) 230-1900
Phone 2: (800) 583-1264
Fax: (405) 230-1903
Email: nami-OK@swbell.net

Oregon
NAMI Oregon
3550 SE Woodward St
Portland, OR 97202-1552
Phone 1: (503) 230-8009
Phone 2: (800) 343-6264
Fax: (503) 230-2751
Email: namioregon@qwest.net

Pennsylvania
NAMI Pennsylvania
2149 N 2nd St
Harrisburg, PA 17110-1005
Phone 1: (717) 238-1514
Phone 2: (800) 223-0500
Fax: (717) 238-4390
Email: nami-pa@nami.org

Puerto Rico
NAMI Puerto Rico
Avenida Andalucia Num. 435
Segundo Piso Urb. Puerto Nuevo
San Juan, PR 00902-2569
Phone 1: (787) 783-6200
Phone 2: (787) 607-4983
Fax: (787) 783-6504
Email: namipr@prtc.net

Rhode Island

NAMI Rhode Island
82 Pitman St
Providence, RI 02906-4312
Phone 1: (401) 331-3060
Phone 2: (800) 749-3197
Fax: (401) 274-3020
Email: nicknami@aol.com

South Carolina

NAMI South Carolina
PO Box 1267
5000 Thurmond Mall Blvd, Ste 200
Columbia, SC 29202-1267
Phone 1: (800) 788-5131
Phone 2: (803) 733-9592
Fax: (803) 733-9593
Email: namiofsc@logicsouth.com

South Dakota

NAMI South Dakota
PO Box 1204
79 Second Street SW
Huron, SD 57350-1204
Phone 1: (800) 551-2531
Phone 2: (605) 352-4499
Fax: (605) 352-5573
Email: namisd@santel.net

Tennessee

NAMI Tennessee
1101 Kermit Dr
Suite 605
Nashville, TN 37217-2126
Phone 1: (615) 361-6608
Phone 2: (800) 467-3589
Fax: (615) 361-6698
Email: sdiehl@namitn.org

Texas

NAMI Texas
Fountain Park Plaza III
2800 South IH35, Suite 140
Austin, TX 78704
Phone 1: (512) 693-2000
Phone 2: (800) 633-3760
Fax: (512) 693-8000
Email: amidad@aol.com

Vermont

NAMI Vermont
132 S Main St
Waterbury, VT 05676-1519
Phone 1: (802) 244-1396
Phone 2: (800) 639-6480
Fax: (802) 244-1405
Email: namivt1@adelphia.net

Virginia

NAMI Virginia
PO Box 1903
One North 5th Street Ste. 410
Richmond, VA 23218-1903
Phone 1: (804) 225-8264
Phone 2: (888) 486-8264
Fax: (804) 643-3632
Email: vaami@aol.com

Washington

NAMI Washington
500 108th Ave NE, Suite 800
Bellevue, WA 98004-5580
Phone 1: (425) 990-6404
Phone 2: (800) 782-9264

West Virginia
NAMI West Virginia
P.O. Box 2706
Charleston, WV 25330-2706
Phone 1: (304) 342-0497
Phone 2: (800) 598-5653
Fax: (304) 342-0499
Email: namiwv@aol.com

Wisconsin
NAMI Wisconsin Inc.
4233 W. Beltline Highway
Madison, WI 53711-3814
Phone 1: (608) 268-6000
Phone 2: (800) 236-2988
Fax: (608) 268-6004
Email: namiwisc@choiceonemail.com

Wyoming
NAMI Wyoming
133 W 6th St
Casper, WY 82601-3124
Phone 1: (307) 234-0440
Phone 2: (888) 882-4968
Fax: (307) 234-0440
Email: nami-wyo@qwest.net

Glossary

activator: a medication that makes a neuron active.

agoraphobia: an irrational fear of leaving the familiar settings of home.

adrenergic receptor: a reactive structural protein molecule on the surface on a neuron that is activated by norepinephrine and/or epinephrine. Two basic types alpha and beta.

alpha receptor: a receptor that is subdivided into two sub-types based on location: alpha 1 located on postsynaptic cell and has stimulating effect. Alpha 2 located on presynaptic cell and has an inhibiting effect.

angioneurotic edema: large circumscribed areas of sudden swelling in the skin usually triggered by allergic reaction. Synonyms giant hives, angioedema.

attunement: the process of sharing non-verbal signals and making fine adjustments in your own mental and emotional state so as to be aligned with those of your child. Such tuning involves changes in eye contact, facial expression, body posture, tone of voice, intensity, timing and rhythm.

axon: the single process of a nerve cell that conducts nervous impulses away from the cell body to another cell.

beta receptor: a receptor that has two major types which generally have opposite and balancing effects. Beta 1 equally sensitive to epinephrine and norepinephrine. Beta 2 100X more responsive to epinephrine.

bulimia: an eating disorder characterized by repeated secretive, uncontrolled bouts of binge eating followed by self-induced vomiting to prevent weight gain.

contingent: the ability of the parent and child to have back and forth signals which are perceived, understood, and responded to. These give and take communications are respectful, and responsive to each other, and result in mutual good feelings.

dendrite: a branching process of a nerve cell that receives nervous impulses and conducts them to the cell body.

dendrite spine: small knobby processes on dendrites where axon terminals closely approach to form a synapse

disease: an illness or disorder of body function characterized by at least two of the following: a recognized cause, identifiable group of signs and symptoms, or consistent anatomic alterations.

d-isomer: molecules with identical chemical composition which exist in two different spatial configurations that are mirror images of each other, are isomers. Two forms exist d (dextro or right sided) and l (levo or left sided)

diagnosis, clinical: a diagnosis made from a study of the signs and symptoms of a disease.

diagnosis, differential: the determination of which of two or more diseases with similar symptoms is the one from which the patient is suffering.

generic: a nonproprietary name as contrasted to the proprietary "brand" name given by pharmaceutical corporations.

hallucination: the apparent, often strong personal perception of an object or event when no such stimulus object or situation is present. The apparent perception can involve hearing, vision, smell, taste, or touch.

holistic: from the viewpoint that a living being must be treated as a complete entity in itself and is more than just the sum of its component parts.

LSD: lysergic acid diethylamide induces visual hallucinations, known as "acid".

MAOI (Type A): monamine oxidase inhibitors (type A) are a class of drug that inhibits the enzymatic oxidation and destruction of monamine (i.e. dopamine, norepinephrine, serotonin) and thereby increase their pharmocologic activity.

narcolepsy: a disorder with involuntary episodes of sleep recurring throughout the day.

neuromodulator: a neurotransmitter that controls the release of other neurotransmitters.

neuron: is the basic unit of the nervous system and functions to conduct electrical stimuli to other cells. It receives multiple inputs from numerous projections called dendrites and send its output by means of a single axon synonym nerve cell.

neurotransmitter: a specific chemical agent released by excitation of a presynaptic neuron into the synaptic space where it moves across to reach the receptor of the postsynaptic neuron.

panic disorder: recurrent panic attacks which have sudden onset, intense fear, and sense of impending doom, accompanied by feelings of depersonalization and unreality.

postsynaptic: referring to the area after the synaptic cleft i.e. postsynaptic neuron (the receiving neuron).

priapism: abnormal persistent and painful erection of the penis which does not result from sexual stimulation and requires emergency medical treatment.

presynaptic: referring to the area before the synaptic cleft i.e. presynaptic neuron (the sending neuron)

prolactin: a hormone produced in the pituitary gland that primarily stimulates the production and secretion of milk but also can inhibit menstruation in females and sexual potency in males.

psychosis: a severe distortion of a person's mental capacity which impairs the ability to recognize reality, to properly interpret sensory perceptions, to think logically, to have appropriate emotional responses, and to cope with the demands of life. Synonym insanity.

psychotropic: capable of affecting the mind, emotions and behavior; denoting drugs used in the treatment of mental, emotional, and behavior disorders.

sign: any abnormality discoverable on examination of the patient that is an objective indication of disease.

stereotypic movements: constant repetition of certain meaningless movements or gestures.

symptom: a departure from normal in the structure, function, feeling or sensation experienced by the patient and indicative of disease.

synaptic cleft: a small space (1-2 trillionths of an inch wide) which separates the sending neuron's axon terminal from the dendrite spine of the receiving neouron.

syndrome: the collection of signs and symptoms describing an illness yet not meeting the criteria of a disease.

terminal, axonal: the club-shaped endings by which axons approach other nerve cells to form synaptic connections.

Some Common Abreviations

ADD	attention deficit disorder
ADHD	attention deficit hyper-activity disorder
BID	twice a day
DSM	diagnostic statistical manual
EPSDT	early periodic screening diagnosis and treatment
FAS	fetal alcohol syndrome
LA	long acting
MAOI	monoamine oxidase inhibitor
MICA	mentally ill chemical abuser
MG	milligram
OCD	obsessive compulsive disorder
ODD	oppositional defiant disorder
PPD	pervasive developmental disorder
PDR	physicians desk reference (for medications)
PRN	when needed
PTSD	post traumatic stress disorder
QD	daily
QID	four times a day
SR	sustained release
SSRI	selective serotonin reuptake inhibitor
TCA	tricyclic antidepressant
TID	three times a day
XR	extended release

QUICK ORDER FORM

Yes, I would like to order
Psychiatric Medications for Children @ $19.95

Ordered by: _____

Send to: _____

Address _____

City _____

State _____ Zip _____

Phone Number _____

Quantity	Unit price	Total
_____	$19.95	_____

Add 6% NJ sales tax
($1.20 for each book)   _____

Shipping for 1 book   3.85

Add $2 for each additional   _____

TOTAL PAYMENT DUE $ _____

SORRY NO CREDIT CARDS OR CASH

Make checks payable to **THE STILLWATER PRESS, INC.**
and mail with completed form to:

The Stillwater Press, Inc. — PO Box 265, Stillwater, NJ   07875
Phone (973) 579–6127   Fax (973) 940-8938